The Scrub's Bible

Richard S. Koplin • David C. Ritterband
Emily Schorr • John A. Seedor
Elaine Wu

The Scrub's Bible

How to Assist at Cataract and Corneal
Surgery with a Primer on the Anatomy of the
Human Eye and Self Assessment

Second Edition

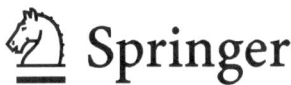 Springer

Richard S. Koplin, MD
Clinical Associate Professor
Co-Director Cataract Division
New York Eye and Ear Infirmary
at Mt. Sinai
New York, NY
USA

Emily Schorr, MD
Associate Professor UNLV School
of Medicine
Shepherd Eye Center
Las Vegas, NV
USA

Elaine Wu, MD
Kaiser Permanente Medical Group
Union City
California
USA

David C. Ritterband, MD
Professor of Ophthalmology
Donald and Barbara Zucker School
of Medicine Hofstra/Northwell
Chief of Refractive Surgery
Manhattan Eye Ear Nose Throat Hospital
New York, NY
USA

John A. Seedor, MD
Professor of Ophthalmology
Donald and Barbara Zucker School
of Medicine Hofstra/Northwell
Chief of Cornea Service
Manhattan Eye Ear Nose Throat Hospital
New York, NY
USA

ISBN 978-3-030-44344-3   ISBN 978-3-030-44345-0   (eBook)
https://doi.org/10.1007/978-3-030-44345-0

This Springer imprint is published by the registered company Springer Nature Switzerland AG
The registered company address is: Gewerbestrasse 11, 6330 Cham, Switzerland

To the indispensable ophthalmic surgical nurses and technicians of the New York Eye and Ear Infirmary—our scrubs—who serve our patients with skill and patience, and rule the operating rooms with grace and humility

The Authors

Contents

Chapter 1
Introduction

In this effort, our second edition of the Scrub's Bible, we have responded to the rapidly changing landscape of innovative technologies and techniques utilized in eye surgery. As in the first edition of the Scrub's Bible, the information is intended for those nurses and technicians who will be attending to operating room procedures in service to modern *ambulatory cataract and corneal surgery*.

Cataract and corneal surgery, including corneal transplantation, are commonly performed safely in hundreds of free standing ambulatory surgical centers around the world – more than 3 million cataract procedures are performed in the United States yearly, virtually all of them performed by the technique known as *phaco-emulsification* with intraocular lens implantation. Modern cataract surgery is one of the most successful operations ever devised, and although technically complex, in the hands of a skilled "*Phaco*" surgeon, the procedure is elegant – even artful.

New and inventive ways to make phacoemulsification more efficient and less complicated – safer – are constantly evolving. Cataract surgery using an ultrafast laser system (**femtosecond laser**) assists in the performance of seminal elements of the procedure without opening the eye. This innovation – using a fast laser in a closed eye environment – is designed to make the surgery more precise, efficient, and – by decreasing the operative time – safer. The challenge is often to make these innovations cost-effective.

Over the past few years, the advances in corneal surgery have been astounding. In many cases total transplantation (penetrating keratoplasty) – the historical standard to rehabilitate an eye with an opaque or distorted cornea – is no longer required. Instead, simply transplanting the inner surface of the diseased cornea – in a short procedure with rapid rehabilitation – will cure a blinding condition. Among other innovations are small plastic polymers that can be inserted into the body of the cornea to refine its shape and thin, microscopic, plastic lenses that are placed within the central cornea to enhance vision.

For the most part what we have provided between these pages is up to date and will serve you well. However, technology and techniques change rapidly, and it is up to you to be inquisitive and preemptive when it comes to maintaining your skills.

© Springer Nature Switzerland AG 2020
R. S. Koplin et al., *The Scrub's Bible*,
https://doi.org/10.1007/978-3-030-44345-0_1

Fig. 1.1 SuperScrub

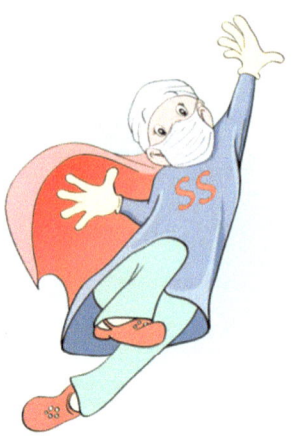

Surgical assisting is a demanding discipline and requires that you be ever atten-
tive to detail. Your lapses may make a relatively easy case difficult for your surgeon
and will sour the OR, not to mention possibly leaving a patient with substan-
dard care.

It is important that you familiarize yourself with each surgeon's technique, style,
and tempo: every surgeon is different, sometimes peculiarly so. Nonetheless, understanding the anatomy and the staging of each part of the procedure unique to that
surgeon and – most importantly – anticipating your surgeon's needs is the difference between an *average* scrub nurse or technician and a *great* one.

As you make your way through the pages of this book, you will occasionally
come across our mascot, *SuperScrub©* (Fig. 1.1). *SuperScrub©* is energetic, full of
dedication to the art of surgical scrubbing, and will highlight some of the information we'll be presenting. We apologize for *SuperScrub's* penchant for putting on a
show; it tends to get restless trapped within the binding of this book all day and is
thrilled you opened it up, freeing it to engage you, even if for a little while.

These are words that virtually every person attached to that area of discipline
understands and are in common usage time and again. Often the words are so commonly used that they develop short forms or vernaculars. (As examples, *phacoemulsification* is "*phaco*," the *anterior chamber* is "the *AC*, and a corneal transplant is a
PK.") These words can be found in the glossary.

Where a word or words are important to the culture of your learning process, it
will be in ***bold and italicized type***. Those words or short forms will be found, as
well, in the glossary of terminology at the end of this book. Become familiar with
these words as part of your new culture.

Chapter 2
The Evolution of Eye Surgery

A Bit of History

As an introduction to the history of eye surgery, consider this: there is almost 5000 years of documented history related to eye care and specifically to cataract surgery – as far back as 2700 BC in Upper Egypt. As you might imagine, across all the subsequent centuries, advances in pharmacology, technology, and techniques did improve outcomes, and now, in the twenty-first century, the promise to restore natural vision has pretty much been met. But, remarkably, 90% of that progress took place only in the past 60 years!

In the early centuries, the ability to perform eye surgery was understandably inhibited by the lack of magnifying devices, small precise operating instruments, medications, and an understanding of sterility and a sophisticated understanding of the anatomy of the eye. Medicines – anti-infective agents and anti-inflammatory preparations in particular – were mainly associated with plant materials and were limited in utility. Available anesthesia was interesting to say the least. A popular form of anesthesia around 500 BC was a combination of potent wine and cannabis (marijuana). Oh, yes, and did we mention the need for restraints at surgery? (See Fig. 2.1).

Remarkably, things changed only marginally for several thousand years. Among early surgeons – or what we might call "proto-surgeons" – some understood that there was something positioned within the pupil that could obstruct vision. Our proto-surgeons were assisted in this understanding by the occasional appearance of a white cloud within the pupil as the once transparent lens degenerated. This frank change in character of the lens was easily seen within the pupil – even at a distance.

So, how did the proto-surgeon of several thousand years ago deal with this degenerated, opaque lens, visible to even a passing observer? Well firstly, and consistent with our unique DNA, our ancestors endeavored to give the phenomenon a qualifying name. You might be familiar with medicine's peculiar penchant for associating medical findings with other natural phenomena. For example, when a

Fig. 2.1 Drawing of patient in restraints late sixteenth century. Georg Bartisch (1535–1607) German physician. (Source: US National Library of Medicine. Image in public domain)

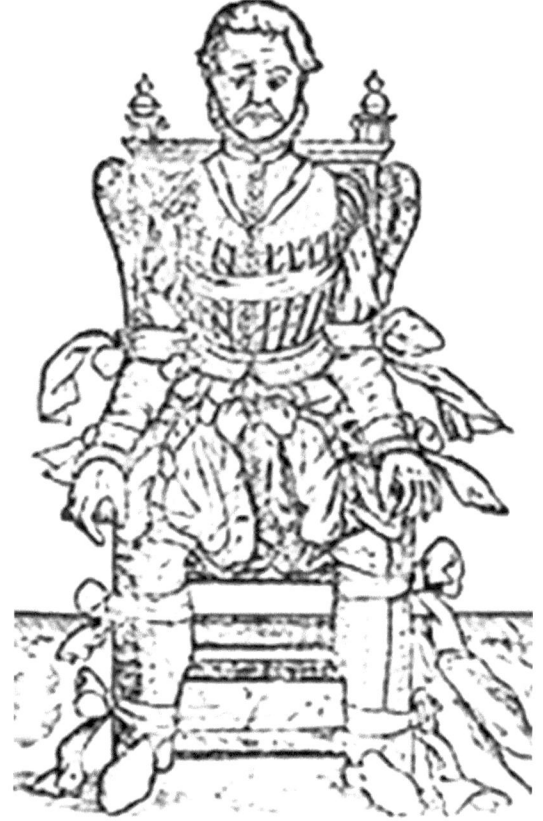

Man restrained for eye surgery
from "Augendienst"
by G. Bartisch (1535-1606)

surgeon studies a tumor, they might describe it as "pea size," or exhibiting a "sponge-like" consistency. A varicose vein might be described as "spiderlike" in appearance.

It seems that our ancient proto-surgeons noticed that the white appearance of a clouded lens within the pupil in those afflicted with blindness was like the turbulent water, foaming white and cascading over a waterfall (Fig. 2.2a). Waterfalls were known to the ancient Greeks as *kataraktes*. So, there you are – white waterfall conflated early on with a degenerated human lens – and by the fifteenth century, the word **cataract** had become the official moniker for a clouded lens, no matter what its state (Fig. 2.2b). So, if you ever take a cruise down Egypt's Nile River, keep your "eye" out for the crashing cataracts that might turn your vacation into a soaking nightmare.

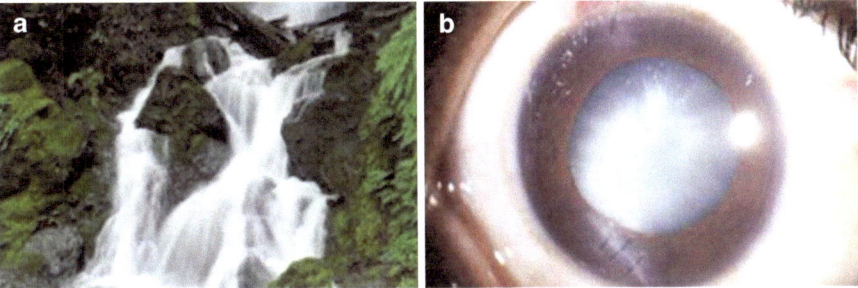

Fig. 2.2 (**a**) Waterfall (**b**) white cataract

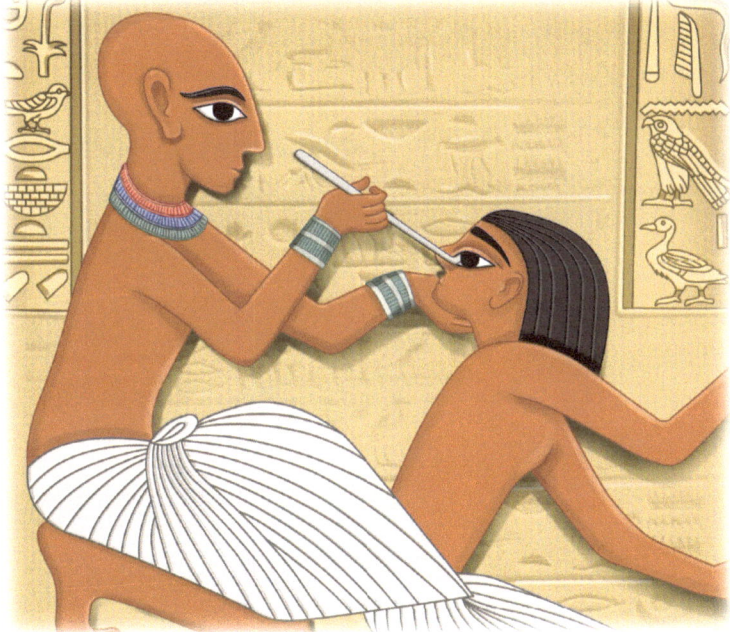

Fig. 2.3 Based on a stone carving of an early cataract surgery circa 200 BC

Now back to our proto-surgeons. How did they respond to the challenge of blinding cataracts in their patients? Without sophisticated surgical tools, ingenuity was key, and although the earliest techniques to cure blindness associated with cataracts would not be considered elegant, they did prove effective – up to a point.

The tomb of King Khasekhemwy, buried in Egypt around 2700 BC, revealed copper tools used to perform a *needling* procedure of cataractous lenses (Fig. 2.3). The needle was inserted into the front of the eye and then used to disrupt the lens and clear it from the pupillary center. This technique and variations became known as *couching* and eventually could be found in common use throughout the Middle

East at the time. The object was to dislocate the lens from its moorings (*zonules*) and push it into the back of the eye and out of the way of the visual axis. (And that is the relationship to the word *couching* which is a French derivation of a word meaning to lie down.)

Look at this drawing from the sixteenth century. We get the chills just thinking about these techniques and the common aftermath, which no doubt included a considerable number of infections, intense inflammatory responses, retinal detachments, and ultimately blind, painful eyes; and not much changed in the subsequent several thousand years. It is well documented that two of history's preeminent composers, Handel and Bach, were blinded by cataract procedures in the eighteenth century.

Now consider that couching – or some variation – was the norm in many parts of the world for almost the next 2000 years (Fig. 2.4). It was performed routinely in third world countries through the twentieth century and is still practiced in certain parts of remote, tribal Africa.

Fig. 2.4 Couching. Georg Bartisch (1535–1607) German physician. (Source: US National Library of Medicine. Image in public domain)

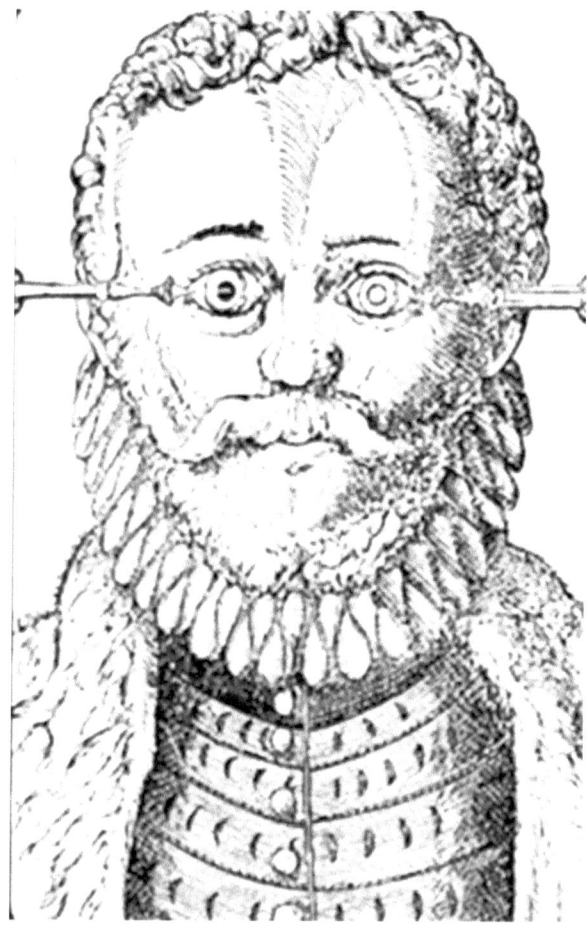

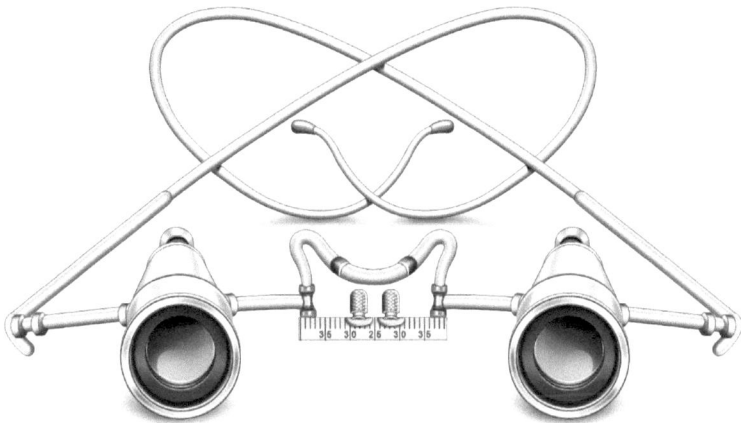

Fig. 2.5 Loupes

Seeing what you're doing at surgery certainly helps, particularly when the anatomic structures are small and often only partially visible. A significant advance took place in the late nineteenth century when magnifying eyeglasses (surgical *loupes* (Fig. 2.5), not unlike those used by jewelers) were introduced to provide an optical assist at surgery.

The ability to visualize the operative field under higher magnification, while simultaneously having a better understanding of the anatomy, provided incentive to revolutionize the treatment of cataracts. From the late eighteenth and early part of the twentieth centuries, western medicine began a slow crawl toward more sophisticated techniques to cure cataracts. Around 1748 *extra*capsular removal of a cataract (***ECCE***) was introduced: the front of the lens capsule – a sort of glassine envelope surrounding the lens – was torn open and its contents washed from the eye, leaving the remainder of the ***capsular bag*** relatively intact (this concept would come in handy 200 years later when lens implantation was introduced). In 1753 a procedure where the entire lens was removed was introduced (*intra*capsular cataract extraction or ***ICCE***). Remarkably, ECCE and ICCE were the mainstay of cataract surgery until the late 1960s – almost 200 years of limited surgical evolution.

Both techniques evolved before adequate small caliber suture materials were in routine use. Silk sutures were first used in 1867, but these were bulky, thick materials and not well suited to eye surgery. Exquisitely thin sutures of nylon material (officially defined by the United States Pharmacopeia as 9-0, 10-0, and 11-0 caliber: the higher the number, the thinner the suture) appropriate to eye surgery would not be in common use until the late 1970s when microscopic eye surgery began to evolve. Prior to the 1970's surgical openings, half the circumference of the cornea was standard for cataract surgery. Without secure wound closure patients would remain in a hospital bed for 5–6 days, their heads "sand bagged" so they would not accidentally turn onto the operated eye. Of consequence, also, was the fact that until the middle of the twentieth century, effective antibiotic eye drops were not available, nor were anti-inflammatory medications: both steroid based and nonsteroidal (NSAID). Prior to the 1970's–1980's a cataract procedure was an unwelcome event among both patients and eye surgeons, and for good reason: the complication rate was high and even a successful procedure left eye patients with uniformally sub-par functional vision.

So, let's assume your patient suffering from a cataract underwent a successful operation. Before the invention of eyeglasses, patients undergoing any type of cataract procedure were damned to a life of severely blurred vision. Removing the crystalline lens of the eye and then failing to replace it leaves the patient in what is called an *aphakic* condition; this is akin to a *camera without a lens*. (*Phakic* means an eye having a lens.) In an aphakic condition objects in view would not be focused on the retina at any distance and therefore vision would be essentially without focus, leaving a patient severely functionally impaired. Vague and ghostly images were all that a patient could expect to experience. Nonetheless, as the only option, it was better than being completely blind.

Crude glasses first evolved in northern Italy (near Venice) in the 14th century when two magnifying lenses, one upon the other, were riveted together and adopted to a mechanism to hold them by hand, or upon the nose, and eventually on frames supported by one's ears (after all that's what ears are for).

The extremely high prescription required to relieve aphakic vision was terribly unnatural, and from the edges of the field of vision, images literally "jumped" into view only to disappear as strikingly to the other side. The character of vision made the patient dysfunctional for many activities. The advent of contact lenses in the mid-twentieth century solved much of those concerns. The thin plastic lenses applied directly to the cornea normalized the image size, but for many elderly individuals – the age of many cataract patients – attempting to manipulate a small, thin piece of plastic and place it securely on the eye was frustrating and at times dangerous.

In the 1970s and 1980s, there was a rapid series of developments. Antibiotic eye drops and ointments, as well as cortisone based and nonsteroidal anti-inflammatory (NSAID) derivatives evolved. Small caliber synthetic sutures were part of the advent of the use of polymers in medicine. The operating microscope with foot control for fine focus and magnification made loupes a thing of the past, and this ability to define the small anatomic elements of the eye introduced the era of *microsurgery*. Suddenly, the entire playing field that was to become modern cataract surgery began to come together: appropriate medications and enhanced visibility led this charge. In the latter part of the twentieth century, medical technology experienced explosive innovation. New devices and the advent of lens implantation were poised to deliver rapid rehabilitation of the cataractous eye with the promise of natural vision.

Some advances in medicine are born of serendipity and at first views seemingly only distantly related to a felicitous outcome. Cataract surgery experienced one of those moments.

It was during World War II that a British eye surgeon (Harold Ridley) noticed that fighter pilots returning from combat with eye injuries that included small pieces of plastic within the eye – the result of shattered plastic canopies machine-gunned by enemy pilots – were relatively free of inflammation. He surmised that the purified plastics used in the canopies were biologically inert – meaning they did not challenge the human immunology system. After the war Dr. Ridley developed a miniature plastic lens which he implanted in several eyes at the time of cataract surgery (c1954). There were still technical challenges to be overcome, but this was a momentous development and would forever change a rather gross and problematic attempt to cure cataracts and restore natural vision, into a sophisticated and highly successful procedure. Lens implantation freed the patient of the burdensome, thick glasses required after surgery and the resulting problematic, aphakic vision. So, eye surgery entered the era of the ***intraocular lens implant (IOL)***. And yet, the operation still consisted of a large incision, multiple sutures, anesthetic injected deep into the orbit, and the need for control of bleeding (hemostasis). What would it take to solve the puzzle of small incision surgery?

In the late 1960s the final piece of the technological challenge was met successfully when a quixotic and inventive eye surgeon by the name of Charles Kelman was sitting in his dentist's chair. If you've ever had your teeth cleaned with modern dental instrumentation, then you have no doubt experienced the very phenomenon that stoked Dr. Kelman's imagination: having your teeth cleaned of plaque and tartar by the *ultrasonic needle* (vibrating at a very high frequency) universally used by most dentists. Dr. Kelman adapted this device in a handpiece to ultrasonically break up (emulsify) a cataractous lens and aspirate (draw out) the liquified lens (an emulsate) from the eye. And Dr. Kelman named it "phacoemulsification" (phaco, or fako, derived from the Greek word for lens and emulsification which grossly means to turn a material into microscopic pieces and mixed with fluid – an emulsion). Phacoemulsification is the gold standard for cataract surgery in most of the developed world. The rest, as they say, is history.

But, not so fast. Phacoemulsification as a revolutionary new procedure – its handpiece, foot-pedal controls, monitoring of a central console to control ultrasonic energy (cutting), fluid infusion, and aspirations: and all managed while the surgeon peers through an operating microscope – was *not* any easy technology to master. The learning curve was (and still is) steep, and many physicians shied from adding it to their skill base. It took more than 25 years of technological improvements – and several resident surgeon generations – to bring Dr. Kelman's device to universal acceptance among surgeons worldwide. Today virtually all cataract surgeons use phacoemulsification in western medicine. With the evolution of phacoemulsification surgeons no longer require a large entry wound into the eye (perhaps 3/4 of an inch or more); now procedures are commonly performed through an incision less than 3 mm – just barely 0.20 of an inch—giving opportunity to avoid suture closure of the wound and using only topical (eye drop) anesthesia.

Modern cataract surgery is often performed in less than 10–15 minutes with the patient spending less than 2 hours in an ambulatory facility, returning home with few restrictions, and perhaps able to return to work the following day. Postoperatively there is usually little inflammation, and vision is rehabilitated rather quickly.

Likewise, corneal surgeons have experienced remarkable improvements in techniques and technologies. Unlike cataract surgery, however, surgery of the cornea has a much more recent history.

The first corneal transplant took place in the early 1900s in what is now Czechoslovakia. Like the historical arc of cataract surgery, but perhaps without the drama of unique devices like surgical ultrasound (phacoemulsification), specific technological and pharmacological needs had to be met. Among these were the operating microscope, fine nylon sutures, sophisticated trephines (a punch-like device to cookie-cut a rounded piece of central cornea – a lenticle – from both donor and recipient to facilitate transplantation), cortisone derivatives (both oral and as an eye drops) to counter the organ rejection, corneal topographic (shape) measuring devices, and other precise imaging tools. Eye banking has made a profound impact on the availability of transplant tissue in the United States and elsewhere. There is rarely a long wait for a donor cornea: perhaps days or several weeks in most cases.

Today, corneal surgeons are also using novel materials to alter the shape and refractive (focusing) properties of the cornea. These prosthetic devices may provide patients with the opportunity to avoid more complex eye surgery in certain cases and, in others, the ability to lessen their reliance on glasses and contact lenses.

Chapter 3
The Advent of Ambulatory Eye Surgery

Modern Day-Op, or *Ambulatory Surgical Centers or Units (ASCs or ASUs)*, are safe and efficient facilitators of both the surgeon's and patient's needs.

An ambulatory surgery center (ASC or ASU) may be independent and owned privately or associated with a hospital, or in some cases there may be a joint venture among doctors and a hospital. When it is part of a hospital complex, the ASC is usually separate and apart from all other operating facilities within that institution (although physically nearby simply to share materials/inventory and manpower).

An ASC is, for the most part, a response to a cost-saving objective where a volume of shorter and less complex procedures can be performed efficiently both in terms of materials and time – *without compromising patient safety*. For this reason, ASCs tend to attract higher-volume surgeons who can maintain high-quality work while performing significant numbers of surgeries in a block time.

The high-volume capacity of an ASC should not interpret this to mean that ASC systems are of lesser quality than the historically less efficient hospital-based systems. A phacoemulsification procedure performed in a well-run independent ASC is usually an extremely satisfactory experience for both the surgeon and patient since there is little wait time and the bureaucratic burden for the patient is significantly lessened.

Hospital ASCs, even when geographically independent from the general hospital operations, often struggle to reach the efficiencies of an independent ASC. The reasons for this may be myriad. Hospital bureaucracies often represent cultures that are difficult to change, unions may have a say in how workers function, and low-volume surgeons – perhaps slower to operate – are more likely to be found in hospital systems than within free-standing ASCs.

In all states ASCs operate under state and federal licensure, and they must conform to well-defined codes, regulations, and standards of operations, identical to the standards imposed on hospitals. It is highly likely that as a scrub tech or nurse, you will be party to a planned or unplanned facility evaluation by a group of state or federal examiners who swoop down on a facility to dissect each detail of its operations. Occasionally there will be scheduled visits from the *Joint Commission*,

© Springer Nature Switzerland AG 2020
R. S. Koplin et al., *The Scrub's Bible*,
https://doi.org/10.1007/978-3-030-44345-0_3

an independent not-for-profit organization that accredits and certifies thousands of programs and healthcare organizations within the United States. Certification by the Joint Commission is recognition that the facility under review has reached the highest levels of quality performance and standards.

These evaluations are stressful to the managing staff as well as to operations since they always take place during the work-day schedule. Your role is to be as supportive as possible and follow the directions of the Medical Director, Chief Nurse, and Facility Administrator of your ASC.

Presurgical clearance from primary care physicians is often *not* a prerequisite to having cataract surgery in a free-standing ASC – assuming the patient's medical issues are stable – while hospital-based systems tend to be conservative by nature and may require clearance and written documentation of a patient's health status.

Not requiring a full presurgical screening evaluation by a primary care physician for entry to a free-standing ASC does not mean that attention to a patient's general medical condition is ignored. A surgeon is expected to be familiar with all aspects of a patient's systemic medical condition, particularly to those issues that might prove to be problematic at surgery. If there is doubt about a patient's medical condition, a full internal medicine evaluation is required, and, in the end, if there is any doubt, it is best to perform surgery in a hospital-based environment matched to the patient's overriding systemic issues.

Cataract surgery and some corneal procedures are considered "minimally invasive," meaning that entry into the eye is uncomplicated by the need for large incisions and is essentially bloodless. Also, these procedures are associated with a low level of complexity, a level that is unlikely to threaten or stress major organ systems – particularly the patient's cardiovascular status. Although there may be some understandable anxiety on the patient's part regarding eye surgery, the intent is to use as little sedation as required to perform a safe procedure. In the main, phacoemulsification surgery for a routine cataract requires only topical anesthesia (eye drops) and often minimal tranquilizing or soporific (drowsiness induced) medications. Blood loss during eye surgery is inconsequential. A retrobulbar injection (an injection of anesthetic below the eye, through the lids and onto the orbit below or above the posterior portion of the eye) is all that is often required for most corneal procedures.

For most patients undergoing cataract surgery within an ASC setting, anesthetics and analgesics are used only briefly – a period of time often measured in minutes – and therefore patients are expected to leave the surgery center alert and fully oriented.

Many cataract surgeons are relative minimalists regarding anesthesia and analgesia, preferring to provide topical (eye drop) anesthesia and use calming speech throughout surgery (vocal anesthesia). However, there are some surgeons who feel more comfortable using a retro- or peribulbar injection of anesthetic into the orbit of the operated eye to provide both anesthesia (diminish sensation and avoid pain) and akinesia (temporary paralysis of eye movement).

Among the concerns that the surgeon should consider before choosing an ASC environment for their patient are cardiac, hematologic, and neurological conditions.

Patients with multiple comorbidities (multiple systemic medical conditions of concern) might be best served in a hospital setting.

Patients with Parkinson's disease or other disorders of movement can often be operated upon in an ASC setting, but this should be evaluated carefully. Children, young adults, and patients with diminished mental capacity or volatile personalities require special attention, and although are operated upon in an ASC setting, both surgeon and anesthesiologist may be more comfortable in a hospital setting.

Occasionally a large ASC (especially if it is multispecialty) may employ an "in-house" primary care physician to perform medical clearance. However, many ASCs utilize their anesthesiologist to provide medical clearance for their patients. In this case the anesthesiologist will take a medical history, evaluate an onsite EKG, and if comfortable with the patient's status then provide analgesia and anesthesia (perform a peribulbar block, if requested by the surgeon), as well as monitor vital signs before, during, and after surgery.

Most importantly, the anesthesiologist is expected to maintain the patient's vital signs and general state of medical equilibrium during the procedure so that they experience minimal stress and report a comfortable experience. If successful, the surgeon will also likely enjoy the experience as well.

Chapter 4
The Eye and Its Anatomical Considerations

Orbit, Lids, and Extraocular Muscles

The eye itself is neatly housed in a protective anatomical structure called the boney *orbit*. It is "cave-like," and the globe (eyeball) sits inside this housing supported by fat and various fibrous septae (think of these as thin-walled tissue compartments that help stabilize an organ like the eye). The eye is well protected from trauma by the bony brow and eyelids.

Extraocular muscles are six thin muscles attached to the outside of the eye at various strategic locations – mostly toward the front of the eye, but invisible to routine inspection – and then attach far back to the boney orbit (Fig. 4.1). They function to allow the eye to move in all directions. Among the disorders affecting muscle movement (motility) are localized disruptions of nerves or blood vessels, stroke, thyroid conditions, neurologic disorders, and trauma. A periorbital injection of an anesthetic agent at cataract surgery is meant to cause temporary immobility

Fig. 4.1 Globe with extraocular muscles

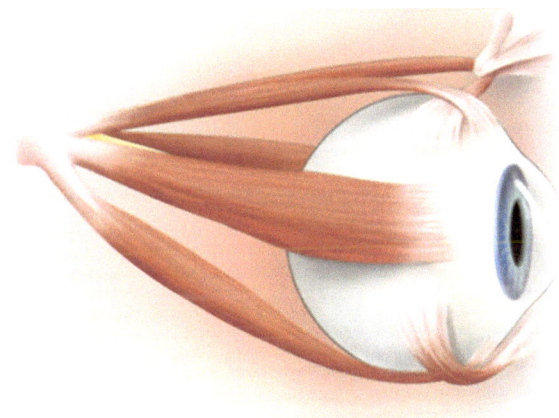

© Springer Nature Switzerland AG 2020
R. S. Koplin et al., *The Scrub's Bible*,
https://doi.org/10.1007/978-3-030-44345-0_4

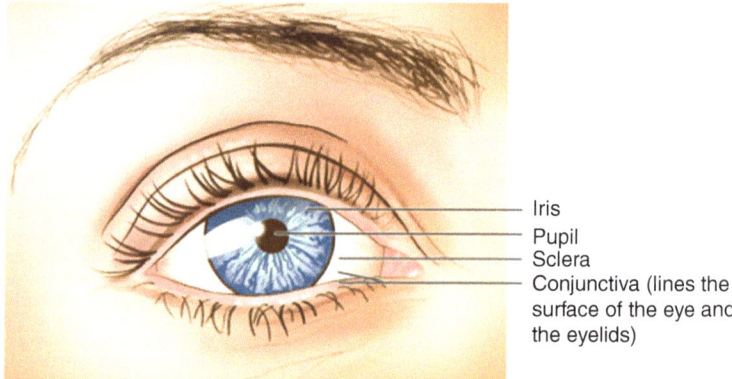

Iris
Pupil
Sclera
Conjunctiva (lines the
surface of the eye and
the eyelids)

Fig. 4.2 Conjunctiva, sclera

(paresis) of the extraocular muscles. This provides reassurance to the surgeon that the patient will not inadvertently move their eye during the procedure.

Rarely, an injection of anesthetic may result in a prolonged temporary or permanent paralysis of an extraocular muscle. This may result in double vision (diplopia).

The *eyelids* perform several functions. Besides being protective, by blinking they sweep tears around the front surface of the eye keeping it moist. The lids contain accessory tear and lubricating glands (meibomian) and help protect the eye from infection and drying (desiccation).

Conjunctiva, Sclera, and Tear Film

The white of the eye (*sclera*) is protected by a transparent tissue: the ***conjunctiva*** (Fig. 4.2). That you can't see the conjunctiva does not diminish its importance to the health of the eye. It is a first line of defense where infection and trauma are issues and its health is important to comfort and visual function. (When your eye gets red, it is mainly the vessels in the conjunctiva that are reacting.)

The ***sclera*** visible at the front of the eye as well as the inner surface of the lids is completely covered by the conjunctiva.

Tears are produced by the ***lacrimal gland*** hidden beneath a bone in the temporal orbit (to the side nearest the ear). Tears are drained from the surface of the eye through an opening on the upper and lower lids near the nose (called a *punctum*). The tears travel through a canal along the lid, into the nose where they flow down your throat. (Explains why, when you cry, you taste the salty tears in your mouth and throat.)

Figure 4.3 shows SuperScrub with watering can dousing front of cornea.

Fig. 4.3 SuperScrub with
watering can dousing front
of cornea

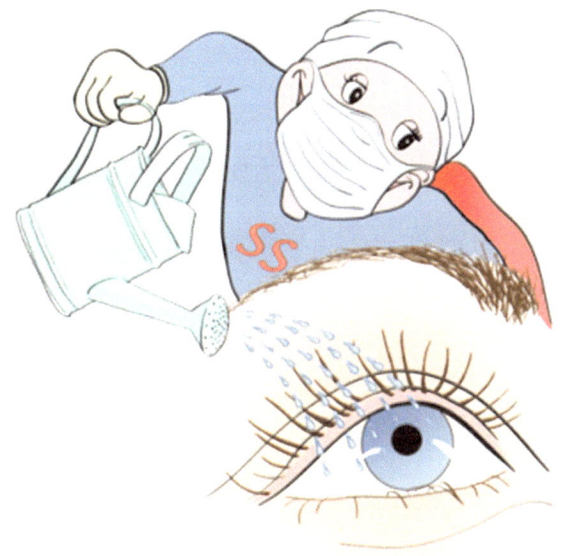

Cornea

The *cornea* is the "window" into the eye. It is a clear tissue that vaults the very front
of the eye and acts as a lens (along with crystalline lens within the eye) and facilitates the transmission of light and images into the inner eye, eventually to reach
the retina.

To provide orientation, if you wear contact lenses, the cornea is where they
would sit. If laser refractive surgery is contemplated (as in Lasik), the cornea is what
is operated upon to effect a refractive change providing you the opportunity to see
without your glasses.

The cornea is a rather resilient, clear tissue that is unique in several ways
(Fig. 4.4).

The cornea is made up of a surface *epithelium* (*the epi*) which is a thin palisade
of cells, protective in nature, and sensitive to its environment. It is easily abraded
(torn) but heals rapidly under most conditions. It sits on a tough membrane
(Bowman's) that acts as platform for the cells to grow.

Abrasions of the epithelium at surgery are commonly seen where surgical prepping is aggressive or where the surgeon might inadvertently strike the eye with a
handheld instrument. The result may be of little consequence to the eventual outcome of the surgery, but postoperatively the patient may have discomfort and some
blurred vision for a day or two.

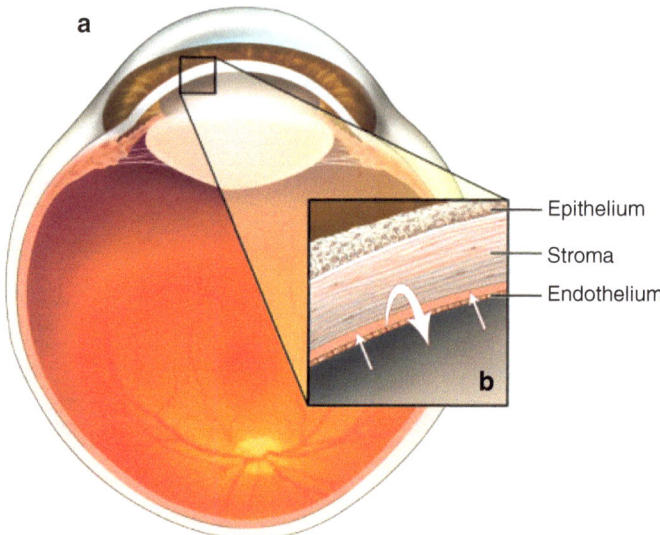

Fig. 4.4 (**a**) Globe, (**b**) corneal layers

The *stroma* of the cornea lies beneath the epithelium and is juxtaposed to Bowman's Membrane; stroma makes up 99% of the corneal thickness. The orientation of the corneal collagen fibers of the stroma is responsible for the efficient transmission of light and images.

A single layer of cells, the *endothelium*, inhabits the entire cornea on the inner surface (inside the eye) which is in direct contact with the fluid (*aqueous*) in the partition known as the *anterior chamber* (*AC*). The endothelial cells are fitted with pump mechanisms. They sit on a clear membrane called Descemet's membrane. Occasionally a surgeon may accidentally partially strip Descemet's membrane during surgery causing a dislocation of the important endothelial cells, resulting in swelling (edema) of the cornea postoperatively, sometimes with permanent ill effect (Fig. 4.5).

Since there is a constant infusion of fluid into the eye through the ciliary body, there is a measurable pressure within the eye (*intraocular pressure or IOP*). Due to this pressure, fluid is constantly being driven into the cornea. If this were to continue unchecked, the cornea would become cloudy and lose the ability to act as a clear window for normal vision.

Even minor trauma to the corneal endothelium during surgery may result in corneal swelling to that portion of the cornea damaged, and the surgeon may commonly note a patch of surface or stromal swelling on the first postoperative visit.

Unique to endothelial cells is their inability to replicate. When traumatized and there is loss of cells, the remaining cells do not split or regenerate to make new cells. Repair to the damaged cornea occurs naturally as the surviving cells grow larger to fill the space where there is loss. Trauma of any sort to the endothelium, including

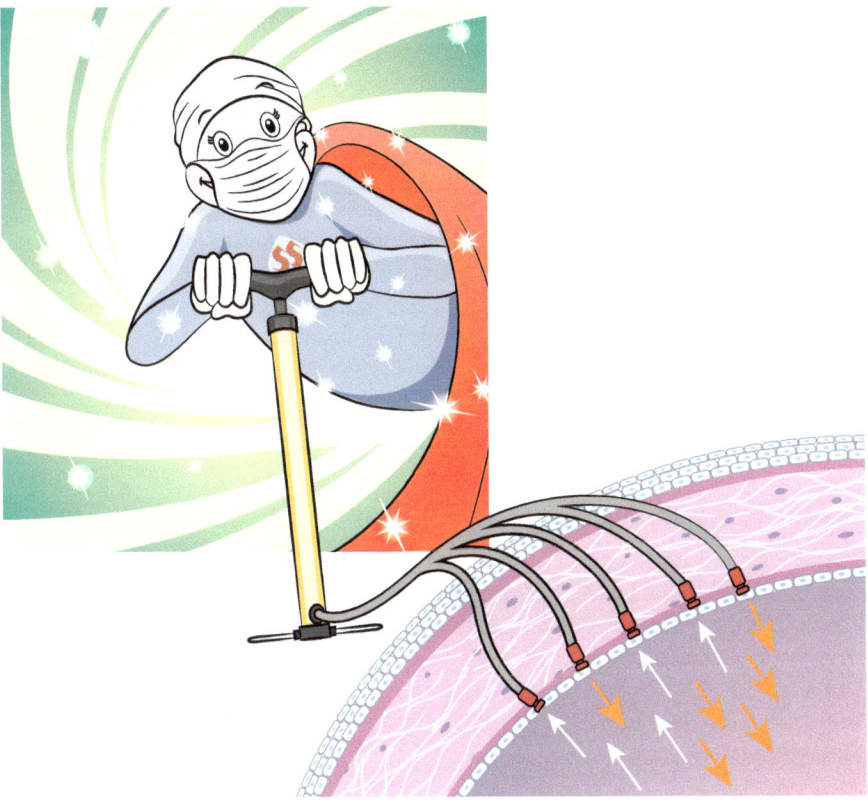

Fig. 4.5 SuperScrub pumping fluid from the endothelial cells of the cornea, returning fluid back into the anterior chamber

excessive infusion of fluid at surgery, toxic drugs, direct trauma, and heat from the phaco-tip, is to be avoided.

Modern cataract surgeons utilize the clear cornea at the far periphery – where it meets the sclera (an area called the limbus) – free of most blood vessels as the ideal area to launch a cataract procedure. Making a small "main" incision (less than 3 mm) with only eye drop anesthesia will provide a micro-eye surgeon with all the room needed to work comfortably within the anterior chamber of the eye while manipulating a phacoemulsification handpiece. An ancillary incision, to the right or left of the main incision (and dependent on the *handedness* of the surgeon), is smaller by half than the main incision and typically 4–5 mm away along the limbus and allows for a bimanual technique (using both hands) to successfully complete a cataract procedure. Most small incision cataract procedures will usually result in a *self-sealing wound* as well as being bloodless, thus the moniker "minimally invasive" surgery.

When a cornea becomes clouded or is irregular in shape, your surgeon will use an entire button of healthy central cornea (epi, stroma, and endothelium) to transplant the diseased cornea. This is known as a penetrating keratoplasty (PK). A

device known as a trephine with a cylindrical blade is used to make a button of central cornea both of the donor and in the recipient; the latter button is disposed of,
while the donor is secured to the recipient using multiple sutures, using a very small
diameter, single filament material (e.g., 10-0 nylon). Often, both single interrupted
and running (like a shoe-lace) are required to fix the donor button securely to a
recipient's eye. You can imagine that securing the donor button in the recipient's
cornea receptacle requires a tremendous amount of skill and patience.

When clouding of the cornea is related to disease of the endothelial cells – where
there are not enough pumps to keep fluid out of the stroma – a DSEK (Descemet
stripping endothelial keratoplasty), or some variation, is often an alternative to a
PK. The surgeon will strip off the patient's Descemet's with its diseased endothelial
cells and replace it with a donor Descemet's with healthy endothelial cells. It's a
simple procedure using a stitchless (suture-less) incision.

Anterior Chamber, Aqueous, and Iris

The *anterior chamber* (*AC*) is that portion of the front of the eye from the inner
surface of the cornea (endothelium) to the *iris* (Fig. 4.6).

The anterior chamber is filled with fluid (*aqueous*) rich in protein, salts, and
oxygen. Since the normal cornea is "avascular" (contains no blood vessels), the
aqueous and tear film are the main source of nourishment and oxygen to
the cornea.

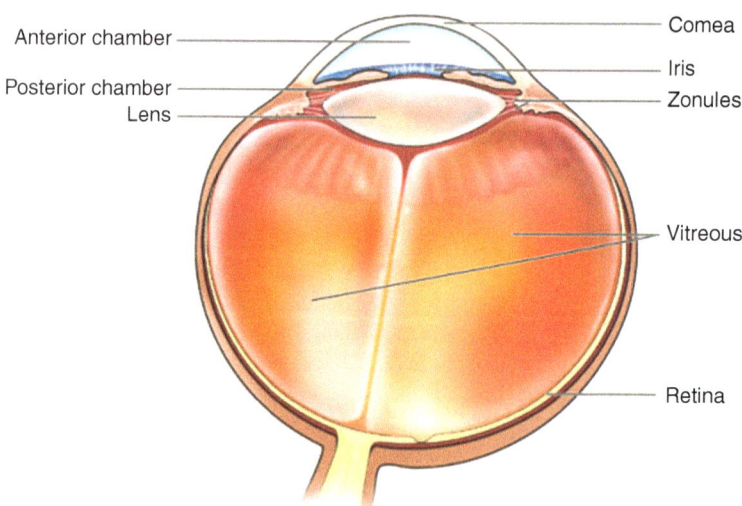

Fig. 4.6 Cross section of anterior and posterior chamber

During cataract surgery, sterile saline fluid is infused into the eye to replace the fluid removed along with the emulsified, cataractous lens. This fluid is designed to be friendly to the endothelium as it replaces the aqueous – at least for the period of the operation. Once the procedure is completed, the eye functions to drain the artificial aqueous from the eye to replace it with the real thing. In a normal eye, this happens in a matter of hours after surgery.

The *iris* is a pigmented, delicate tissue with an opening in the center – the *pupil*. Under normal conditions a thin ring of muscles surrounds the pupil allowing for *dilation* (opens) in low light and *constriction* (becomes smaller or miotic) in bright light. Since the lens lies *behind* the iris, a fully dilated pupil is most accommodating to the surgeon's needs. Certain drugs – as eye drops – are used to facilitate the dilating process prior to surgery.

Posterior Chamber and Crystalline Lens

The compartment located *behind* the iris and filled mainly with the crystalline lens is called the *posterior chamber* (*PC*). It too contains aqueous. The crystalline lens is held in place within the eye by thousands of thin fibers (*zonules*) known as the suspensory ligaments. These micro-thin fibers are attached around the entire lens capsule at its equator and at their far ends are inserted against the inner eye wall (ciliary body). The zonules not only support the crystalline lens securely – and keep it centered – but assist in changing the lens shape to refocus the image on the retina for near vision. This is known as *accommodation*.

In its normal state, the *crystalline lens* is clear as glass and surrounded by its *capsule.* The capsule is a thin glassine-like envelope which is, unfortunately, capable of being breached or torn during surgery. When the lens becomes clouded or discolored, the *entire lens* is simply referred to as a cataract.

Performing a cataract procedure using the phacoemulsification technique requires that the surgeon make a controlled round tear in the front (anterior) capsule of the lens (cataract) known as a *capsulorrhexis* or *rhexis.* This opening is a circumferential (circular) tear designed to avoid small radial nicks or other imperfections since forces applied to the rhexis with nicks during surgery will tend to tear out. This could seriously compromise the procedure. An adequate rhexis is required so that the nucleus – the center of the lens – within the capsule can be approached and removed using a phacoemulsification tool.

Once the nucleus is emulsified and aspirated from the eye, there is still lens material remaining. This is known as cortical lens material and is rather firmly attached to the inside of the intact capsule. The cortex is removed using a second instrument attached to the phaco-console. It is called an irrigation-aspiration (I&A) hand-piece. Loose edges of cortex are captured by the aspiration inflow and carefully drawn into the handpiece. Eventually all the cortex is removed. The capsule, once emptied of all lens material, is then referred to as the "capsular bag" (or just the bag) and is a ready receptacle for insertion of the plastic (acrylic) lens implant (*intraocular lens or IOL*).

Fig. 4.7 SuperScrub
holding up lens
with zonules

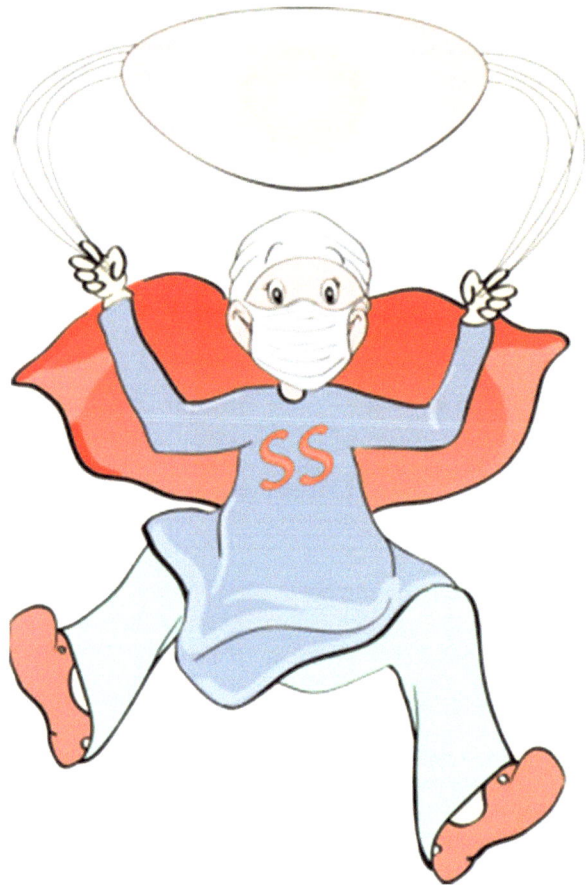

You can imagine that the stability of the zonules is of paramount importance during cataract surgery. If a patient has a disease of the zonules, weakening them, or the surgeon's technique is overly aggressive, there is the potential for the zonules to tear and the lens to fall out of position during or after surgery (Fig. 4.7).

There is an anatomic landmark within the posterior chamber (PC) that is occasionally important to cataract surgeons as they perform their surgery. It is known as the *ciliary sulcus*, and it lies just in front of the insertion of zonules barely in front of the lens, but so far to the periphery that it is hidden from view even with a dilated pupil. It runs ringlike around the entire circumference of the eye. It's sort of a gutter: a place that is empty of any important structures. Because it is free of sensitive anatomical structures, it can be used as an alternative fixation for an artificial lens implant (IOL) if the capsular bag is damaged and cannot support a lens implant. Take note of this anatomic area, since it will be revisited in the section on lens implantation at the time of cataract surgery.

Vitreous Body

Most of the eye behind the lens is filled with a *gelatinous-like* substance known as **vitreous**. The vitreous body acts to cushion the eye and transports nutrients. Although an eye can function without a full complement of vitreous, how vitreous is handed surgically and under what conditions – as a planned or, unhappily, unplanned event requires a bit of explaining.

The vitreous is mobile and is attached rather firmly to the retina in the far periphery, and here is where our respect for the vitreous body is heightened. Untoward movement of the vitreous may cause traction – pulling – most strategically on the retina in the far periphery. Due to the danger of tractional tears occurring to the retina – often threatening a detachment, or separation – any surgery where the vitreous is implicated is best approached by a trained vitreoretinal surgeon. Vitreoretinal surgeons are trained and are comfortable working in a "closed environment," working through several micro-incisions made into the sclera behind the lens (anatomically known at the *pars plana*). The surgeon will employ sophisticated vitreous cutting and aspirating tools (a vitrector) which provides for a stable, controlled operation with minimal traction applied to the retina – a good example is surgery of the vitreous and retina where diabetic proliferative disease is threatening a patient's vision.

On the other hand, an unplanned experience with the vitreous may occur when a cataract procedure goes awry. The event – perhaps a cataract surgeon's most disappointing intraoperative complication – occurs when the surgeon inadvertently breaches the posterior capsule or tears a considerable number of zonules supporting the lens while manipulating the phaco- handpiece of ancillary instruments. In either case the vitreous may spill into the front of the eye (anterior chamber). Implicit in this untoward event is the potential traction on the retina, generating the fear of detachment of the retina in the postoperative period. At surgery the surgeon is usually obligated to use a vitrector through the operative wounds to attempt a cleanup of the vitreous as it spills into the anterior chamber (AC). However, the vitreous is colorless and sneaky in its ability to avoid detection, so the surgeon may find it maddening to completely clear the front of the eye of vitreous strands and the threat of vitreoretinal traction. Where this may occur, your surgeon may request injectable dexamethasone to be introduced into the anterior chamber of the eye. The dexamethasone – milky white – has the remarkable ability to stick to the vitreous gel, assisting in identifying its presence.

Additionally, with the capsule breached, and/or zonules damaged, there is little to prevent cataractous lens material from slipping into back of the eye, far from being easily retrieved. This complication often requires intervention by a vitreoretinal surgeon on the spot or in the days immediately after the surgical misadventure. The technique for removal of errant lens material deep in the eye is known as a pars plana vitrectomy and takes advantage of the anatomical area between the ciliary body and retina – known as the pars plana (where there are no important anatomical considerations) – where instruments such as the vitrector are able to efficiently remove the lost lens material.

Figure 4.8 shows vitreous strands tugging on the retina with hole and detachment.

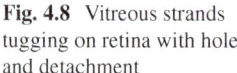

Fig. 4.8 Vitreous strands tugging on retina with hole and detachment

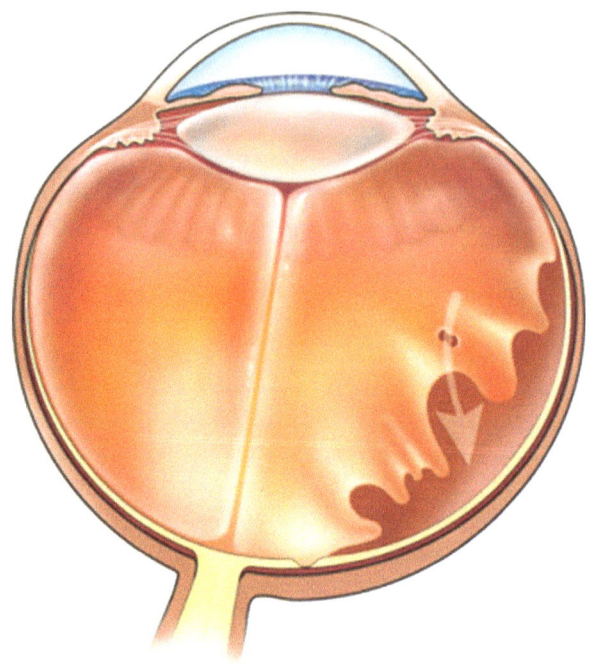

Retina, Choroid, and Optic Nerve

Images passing through the cornea and lens are ideally focused on the retina. The *retina* (Fig. 4.9) makes up the inner wall of the back of the eye and is a broad sheet of tissue containing two types of photoreceptors called rods and cones. *Rods* are responsible for vision at low light levels, while *cones* are responsible for vision at high light levels. Cones are also capable of color vision, while rods are not. The center of retinal function is an area called the macula, and an even more discrete area inside the macula, the fovea, is populated exclusively by cones; a healthy fovea provides the most detailed vision. The fibers from the rods and cones are bundled together into the optic nerve, the beginning of a visual transport system.

Nourishing the deeper (outer) areas of the retina is an extensive spongy tissue called the choroid: a maze of lacunae containing blood, membranes, and erectile tissue (Fig. 4.10).

The retina, however, is not where you "see." Once the cornea and lens deliver an image to the retina, it is only the first stop along an elaborate a transport system.

The *choroid* lies beneath the retina and is a vascular network that nourishes parts of the retina. Its relevance to cataract surgery is the rare instance of bleeding from the choroid that can be catastrophic (*suprachoroidal hemorrhage* or *expulsive hemorrhage*). It is an unusual occurrence and is more common in cataract surgery performed without phacoemulsification, where larger wounds are used and the eye exposed to abnormally low pressures for extended periods during the surgery.

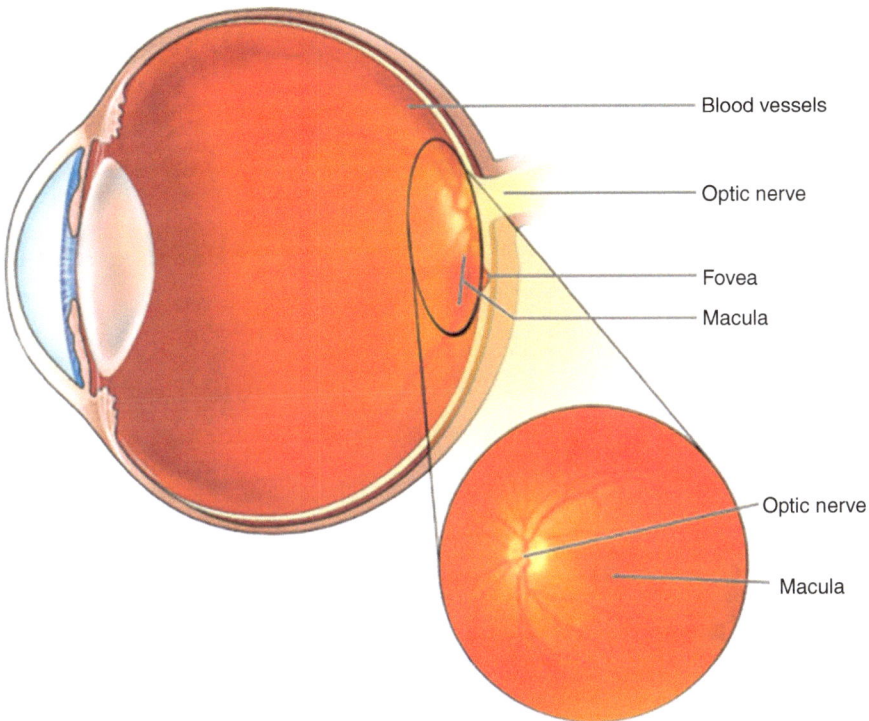

Blood vessels

Optic nerve

Fovea

Macula

Optic nerve

Macula

Fig. 4.9 Retina and macula

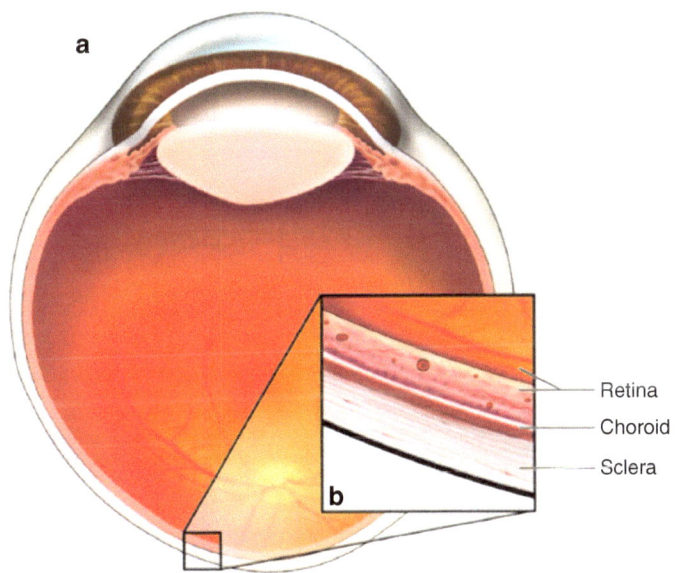

a

b

Retina

Choroid

Sclera

Fig. 4.10 Anatomic details of relationship among retina, choroid, and sclera

Chapter 5
How We See

In looking around, and without conscious effort, your eyes scan and find the "object of desire." Usually that is the object you have consciously determined to be the focus of attention across your field of vision. As example, when you receive your paycheck, your eyes invariably go to the dollar amount in the upper right corner: the object of desire consciously sought out.

The remainder of the check is "appreciated" through the passive nature afforded by your peripheral vision; you know it's there, but the object of interest to you is the amount of the check brought front and center. Your optical-neurological systems have teamed up and have identified the importance of the object of desire and without conscious effort have placed the image on the central retina at an anatomical place called the *macula* (Fig. 5.1).

Once the image is placed central to the macula (within a microscopic area called the *fovea*), it is then bundled along with the peripheral images into the ***optic nerve***

Fig. 5.1 SuperScrub counting money

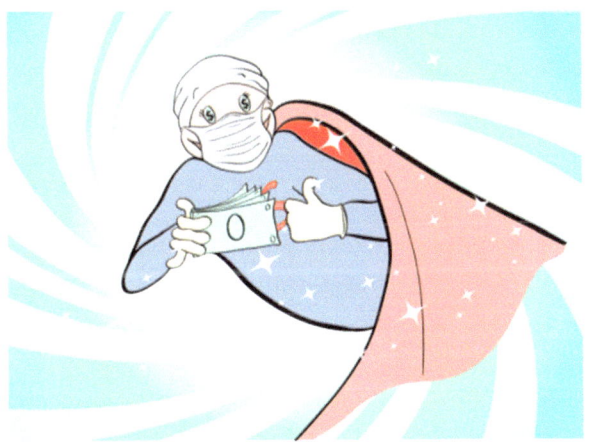

and then trundled along the visual pathway of the brain, eventually to the visual cortex – at the very back of your head (Fig. 5.2). And it is here that there is conscious awareness of "seeing" (Fig. 5.3).

Fig. 5.2 Illustration of image on macula, moving along the optic nerve towards brain

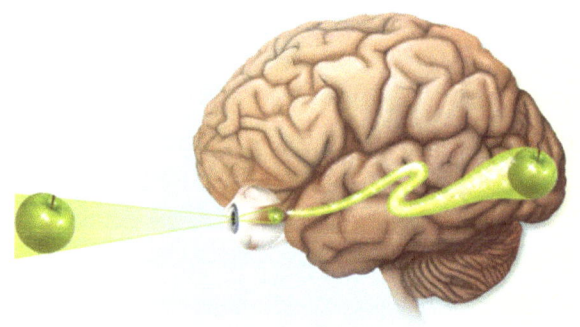

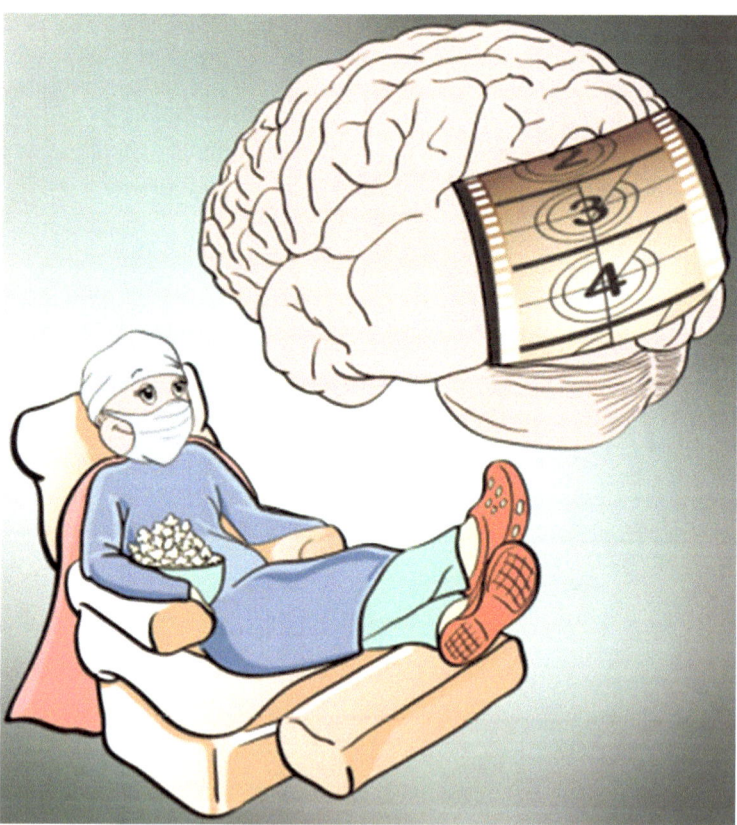

Fig. 5.3 SuperScrub in a lounge chair watching a movie across the occipital cortex

Chapter 6
Contemplating Cataract Surgery

As we've discussed, when the crystalline lens becomes cloudy (or opaque), the lens is then called a cataract. It does not matter exactly where the cloudiness appears within the lens; it is still called a cataract, even if the cloudiness does not interfere with vision.

We define the areas of cataractous lens change within the lens as nuclear where the cloudiness is central, posterior subcapsular when a sandpaper-like cloudiness spreads across the back of the lens and cortical when white cloudy material fills the lens in between the nucleus and the capsule. In fact, a patient can have elements of all three.

When a cataractous lens is left to "mature" for long periods, it may become extremely firm – rock hard, in fact – and dark in color. The result is called brunescence, and when it is even further advanced (hypermature), it may become completely milky white. These advanced lens changes may be challenging to your surgeon and may imply a higher risk of complication, as well as require special techniques at surgery.

Cataracts are often associated with the aging process; however, there are disorders, such as diabetes, that seem to make patients more prone to cataract development. There are children born with cataracts (congenital), and here there is often a strong genetic relationship, so it is not uncommon to find a considerable number of family members with congenital cataracts.

Cortisone is causally related to the development of subcapsular cataracts (sandpaper-looking changes in the back of the lens across the posterior capsule). Smoking, ultraviolet light, and trauma to the eye (including the likes of air bag injuries, penetrating injuries, and previous intraocular surgery) are among other potentially causative agents.

Your surgeon will take note of the type of cataract during their initial preoperative evaluation of their patient in their office and enter the operating room with a pre-planned surgical template based on any number of observations.

Among the considerations your surgeon will likely have taken note of will be the firmness (hardness) of the cataractous lens, the perceived health of the zonules, the size of the eye, the depth of the anterior chamber (need room to manipulate instruments and lens material), the ability to dilate the pupil and keep it dilated, and the health and clarity of the cornea. Finally, the patient's personality and perceived capacity to cooperate will be considered.

Certain oral and topical drugs may have potential impact on your surgeon's ability to perform an uncomplicated procedure. Oral alpha blocking agents (and other drugs in this family), — are oral agents used to treat prostate enlargement and urinary frequency, and may cause the pupil to dilate poorly and then during the operation cause the iris to become annoyingly floppy (intraocular floppy iris syndrome or IFIS) while simultaneously becoming more miotic (smaller). Pilocarpine eye drops, long used in glaucoma treatment until recent years, may make the pupil too small to operate comfortably without the use of devices to extend the diameter of the pupil (iris hooks). (Even many years after stopping the medication).

The surgeon, based on their assessment of the patient, will typically inform the anesthesiologist as well as their scrub of their concerns. A plan will be developed to assure control of the patient during the procedure, and your anticipation of any threat or idiosyncrasy will be extremely important.

Your added value as the surgical scrub will be your ability to understand the various challenges and be prepared to assist your surgeon in anticipating and meeting those challenges. It is always appropriate to query your surgeon to any concerns they might have prior to initiating surgery. This will make you more alert to potential issues that might arise, and it will certainly impress your surgeon.

Why a Patient Undergoes Cataract Surgery

We speak of activities of daily living (ADLs) when we consider recommending cataract surgery to a patient. Each patient's needs differ, and therefore the need for cataract surgery is variable.

A younger, working patient might have greater demands than, say, an 80-year-old patient who has given up driving and lives a sedentary life. On the other hand, we consistently care for patients where 75 is the new 40 and the needs for senior citizens who are golfing, biking, traveling, and working can often be identical to younger patients.

On rare occasions a cataract might be associated with a secondary problem – often called a ***comorbidity***. These conditions may press the patient and surgeon to consider cataract surgery outside of strict visual needs. Examples include a hypermature lens (swollen and possibly leaky) causing inflammation, or an increasing risk of glaucoma due to an enlarging cataractous lens. Also, for diagnostic and treatment purposes, a retinal surgeon may ask the cataract surgeon to consider removing the cataractous lens so that they may better visualize, diagnose, and treat a retinal or choroidal disorder.

So, unless there is a comorbid condition, the surgeon's job is to confirm that any visual changes are related to a developing cataract and counsel the patient in relation to their visual needs (ADL's).

Chapter 7
How the Patient Gets from the Front Door of the ASC to Your OR Suite

The Necessary Bureaucracy

The patient, once arriving at the ASC, will complete paper work at the admitting/ reception desk. These will typically include medical-legal consent forms, financial information, and general instructions. The patient will then be moved to the *pre-op staging area.*

This is an appropriate time to remind the patient to consider going to the toilet.

Often the patient is not required to remove their clothing for surgery, and instead they are supplied with a gown that pretty much covers all of their street clothes. Sterile booties slipped over shoes, and a head cover is placed. The patient is now ready for the prep-stage.

Preoperative Area Procedures

The patient is typically welcomed to the pre-op area by a nurse or nurse extender who takes a medical history, sets up blood pressure and EKG monitors, and confirms the eye to be operated upon. Certain concerns will be immediately addressed.

Patients with latex allergies and those with a history of allergies to certain eye drops will be determined and alerts passed to the surgeon and OR staff. Where the patient is allergic to latex, you should plan on substituting latex-free gloves for all involved with the surgery.

As previously noted blood tests (save for the occasional finger stick for blood sugar) are not routinely performed in free standing ASCs and only occasionally in hospital-based ASCs.

The eye to be operated upon is confirmed by paper work (including a surgeon's preadmission note) as well as verbally by the patient.

© Springer Nature Switzerland AG 2020
R. S. Koplin et al., *The Scrub's Bible*,
https://doi.org/10.1007/978-3-030-44345-0_7

Prior to moving a patient to the OR, the surgeon must again confirm the eye to be operated upon by placing their initials (or other proscribed identifying mark) on the forehead just above the eye to be operated with an indelible soft pen. The entire staff should be very compulsive regarding assuring themselves which is the correct eye to operate upon. Don't assume that the patient knows!

At some point prior to moving the patient from the preoperative area to the OR, the patient will be introduced to the attending anesthesiologist. Although the anesthesiologist's expectations are that the surgeon has performed an assessment of the patient's capacity to undergo outpatient cataract surgery, he will nonetheless further review the patient's general medical status. This will include discussing medications routinely used and possible drug allergies. The anesthesiologist will also assess the patient's emotional state.

The surgeon will be apprised by the anesthesiologist of any concerns. For instance, during the pre-op evaluation, the anesthesiologist may note that the patient's blood pressure is somewhat elevated. The anesthesiologist might suggest a short-acting hypertensive medication be used to bring the pressure down prior to initiating the procedure.

There may be times when a patient's blood pressure is inordinately high, and the anesthesiologist will recommend cancelling the case. The surgeon will generally follow the admonitions of the anesthesiologist.

Another example of concern is a cardiac arrhythmia. Here again the surgeon will be very respectful of the anesthesiologist's concerns and will follow their lead in canceling the case. In some cases the anesthesiologist will wish to speak with the patient's personal physician, and in rare cases where there is a life-threatening finding (usually blood pressure or cardiac related), the anesthesiologist might insist that the patient go directly to the emergency room.

If all is well, and the anesthesiologist has pronounced a patient competent for surgery, the nursing staff will continue the initial prep of the patient, while they are still in the pre-op area. This will include instillation of dilating eye drops – usually *tropicamide* and *neosynephrine* (occasionally, along with a topical anesthetic).

Depending on the surgeon's habits, several drops of an *antibiotic* will be applied to the designated eye to be operated, along with a *nonsteroidal anti-inflammatory* drug useful in maintaining dilation and decreasing discomfort.

At the proscribed time, the patient will then be moved to the operating suite where they will be placed on an operating table and a reconfirmation process is once again begun.

Chapter 8
Decorum in the OR

Often overlooked in the OR suite is the practice of appropriate decorum – especially once a patient has arrived in the suite. Any music playing should be turned off unless otherwise requested by the surgeon or patient. Laughing and telling jokes or speaking of personal matters should be avoided in the presence of a patient. Do not discuss complications that might have occurred to a previous patient and do not make disparaging remarks about anyone.

All attention should be given to the patient, their comfort and safety, as well as to the expert setup for the procedure to begin shortly. Speak directly to the patient, ask how they are feeling, and inquire if there is anything you can do to make them more comfortable. Pay attention to head positioning: the head should be level with the floor and not angulated up or down; this prevents the eye itself from sitting in an unacceptable position for the surgeon.

Do not bring cell phones or other personal electronic devices into the operating area.

In all cases think what you would want to hear in the OR while being prepared for an anxiety-provoking operation. Treat the patient as you would wish to be treated!

And lastly, used caps, gloves, and boots are not toys and should be disposed of properly (Fig. 8.1).

© Springer Nature Switzerland AG 2020   33
R. S. Koplin et al., *The Scrub's Bible*,
https://doi.org/10.1007/978-3-030-44345-0_8

Fig. 8.1 SuperScrub with a surgical glove blown up over its head

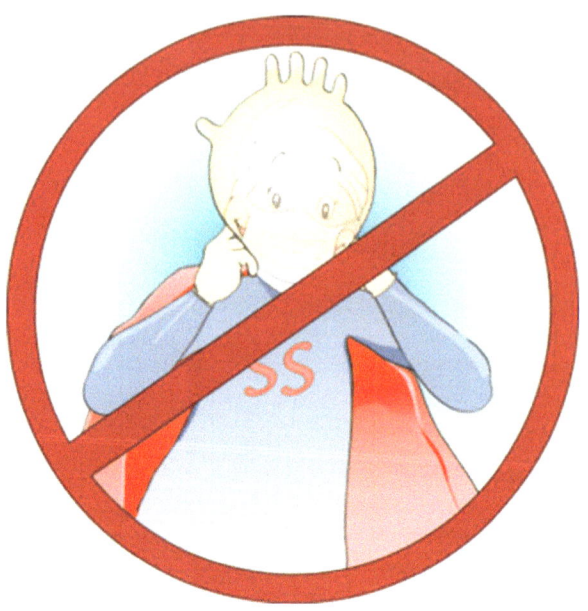

Chapter 9
Infection Control

Despite which individual is responsible for actually cleaning and initiating the sterilization of your surgical instruments (and depending on the habits of the ASC, this might be the scrub just finishing a case or a designated individual with a specialized function), everyone associated with the operating room is part of the *infection control team* and is responsible for maintaining the integrity of sterile procedures.

Operating caps, boots, and clean scrub suits (Fig. 9.1) are to be worn in the area delineated at the operating rooms and inclusive hallways. And anyone leaving the

Fig. 9.1 SuperScrub in scrub suit

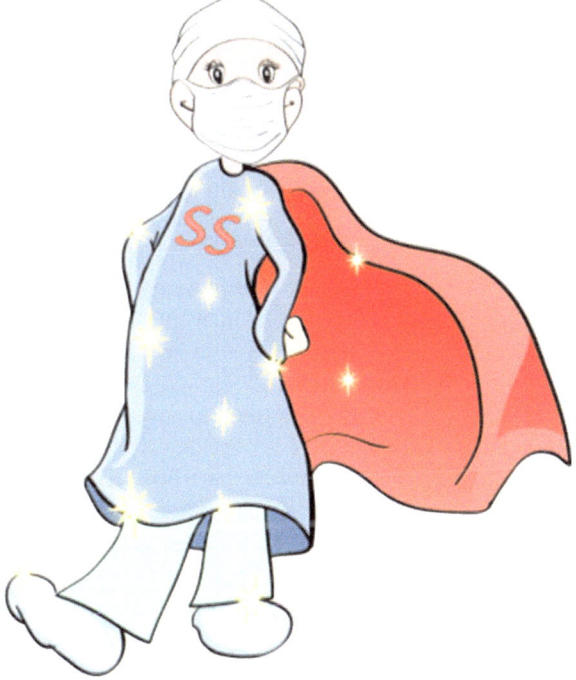

ASC itself should remove their scrubs and change into clean scrubs, boots, and caps on return.

IF AN EMPLOYEE OR SURGEON LEAVES THE ASC IN A SCRUB SUIT AND RETURNS, THEY MUST ONCE AGAIN CHANGE INTO A FRESH SCRUB!

Operating rooms – both hospital and free standing – generally function under state and federal regulations and oversight. The Occupational Safety and Health Administration (OSHA) publishes guidelines directed at controlling exposure to pathogenic microorganisms in the workplace. ASCs post the most salient elements of these guidelines in a prominent place in the center. Additionally, various state Departments of Health's (DOHs) will express wide control over an ASC's operation – some states seemingly more aggressive than others. It's amazing, when it comes to infections control, what objects may become the focus of at DOH's attention. Consider the lowly and seemingly insignificant garbage pail and how its cover is opened and closed. No hands, please, foot controls rule! And when you think about it, it certainly makes sense to keep your hands far from waste materials.

Adequate cleaning and sterilization of instruments – and the maintenance of sterile procedures – are the single most important objectives among operative concerns in your center. *Breaks in sterile technique cannot be tolerated!* Any lapses must be corrected immediately, and every individual involved in the operating emporium must consider corrective actions to perceived concerns. Managing the operating suites is a *team commitment.*

Instrument Cleaning

A typical cleaning and sterilization procedure might be as follows:

Instruments are brought directly to the "clean room" from the OR suite after a surgical procedure. This is a room large enough to contain one or several autoclaves (sterilizing systems) as well as sinks for pre-cleaning instruments prior to sterilization.

Instruments are handled one at a time and washed with tap water. Do not "gang" wash instruments since many instruments are delicate, and banging them into one another can cause damage. Do not use salt water (saline) to clean instruments.

Delicate hand instruments should be gently brush cleaned, but aggressively enough to free any detritus (debris) caked on them. Any blood or lens material that remains on instruments will become solidly "bake on" by the sterilization process, and although this may not be a sterility issue (although it may be), the finding of human material on a presumably clean instrument at surgery is, if nothing else, off putting.

Just prior to sterilization, instruments are examined for damage under a table-stand magnifying glass. The examiner should reject any instrument that is bent, missing teeth, or out of alignment. Damaged and dirty instruments (Fig. 9.2) – and this includes instrument with rust particles – should not find their way to the operating table.

Fig. 9.2 Damaged
instruments.
(Photographer:
Bob Masini)

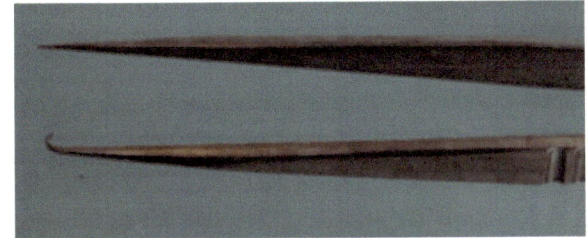

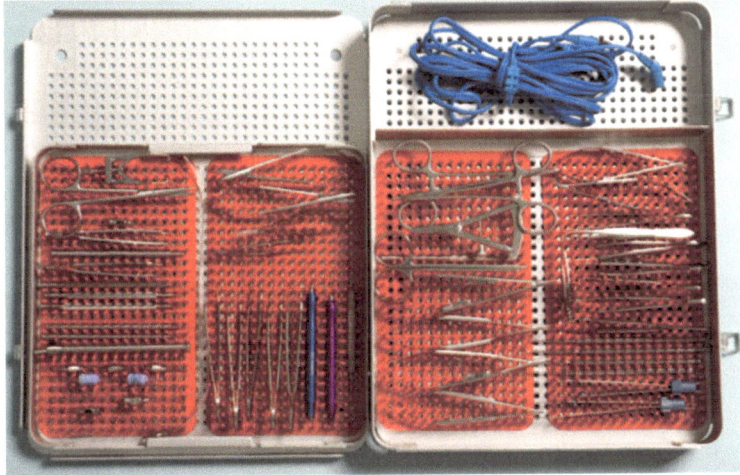

Fig. 9.3 Open instrument caddy. (Photographer: Bob Masini)

Special attention is to be given to the inner tubular portion of the phaco and I&A handpieces (where fluid runs in and out). After each surgical procedure, these instruments should be forcefully flushed with warm water under high pressure using a 3cc syringe. Any material remaining (such as lens debris) in a metal tubular instrument once thoroughly baked on will cause a blockage to fluids meant to flow freely. This will be frustrating to your surgeon and could be dangerous.

Instruments are then placed in a metal or heat-resistant acrylic instrument caddy containing a silicone or composite pronged mat to keep instruments from moving and damaging one another (Fig. 9.3). The instrument caddy is then placed in the appropriate sterilizer.

Sterilization

Two methods of sterilization are used in most surgery centers. These are autoclave (steam under pressure) and gas (usually ethylene oxide) systems. The system in use at your ASC should be thoroughly explained to you.

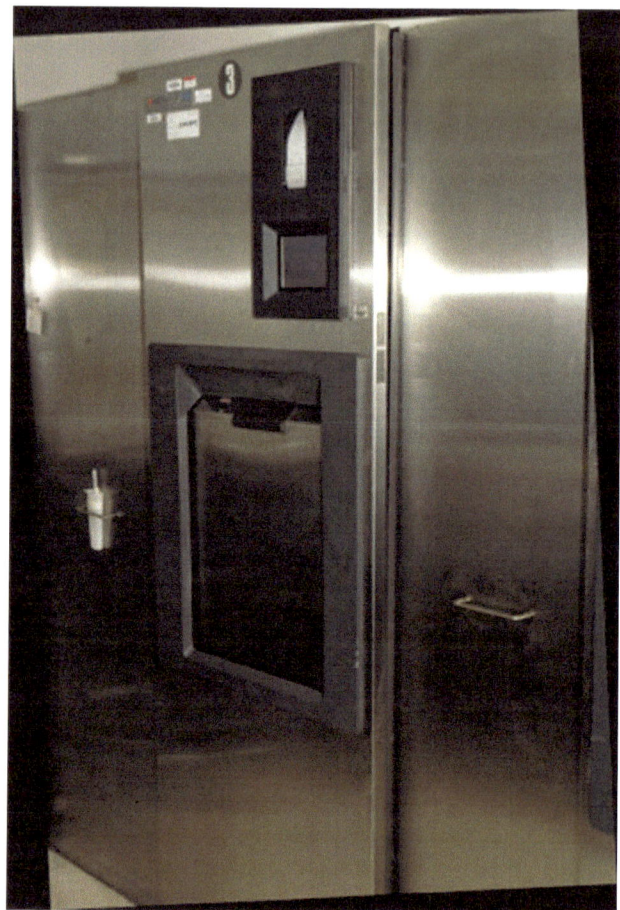

Fig. 9.4 Steam autoclave. (Photographer: Bob Masini)

Since *moist heat* is more efficient in killing microorganisms than dry heat, a steam autoclave (Fig. 9.4) working at 15–20 pounds of pressure at 250° for approximately 30 minutes is a standard. At higher temperatures, the sterilization cycle may be as little as 3 minutes. The latter is often called *flash sterilization* and is usually reserved for the sterilization of a single instrument needed for immediate use.

Gas sterilization uses ethylene oxide, and although less traumatizing to stainless steel and titanium instruments, it takes an inordinately long time (up to 2 hours). One rarely finds a gas sterilizer in an ophthalmic ASC since the turnaround time from case to case requires rapid reuse of surgical instruments. To use a gas sterilizer in an ophthalmic ASC, one might require 4–6 full surgical instrument trays available each morning per room: expensive and not very practical.

After sterilization, instruments are delivered to the OR suite still in their sterile caddies. Once opened by the *unsterile* circulating nurse/technician, you will carefully remove the instruments to your sterile instrument table. The instruments, if fresh from the sterilizer, are then allowed to cool. Once cooled, you will begin to assemble the various instruments across the table.

The scrub's instrument table is usually a stainless steel cart on wheels measuring approximately 4–5 feet by 2.5 feet. It is draped with sterile paper coated with a plastic surface. This lessens the population of small pieces of microscopic paper thread and fine paper dust finding their way into the eye along with instruments.

In between cases, the OR suite will be cleaned of the litter from the previous surgery. This chore will include mopping up water and other fluids spilled to the floor and picking up small sponges, needles, syringes, as well as paper and plastic containers that may have been dropped.

The patient operating table itself is examined for debris and damp spots which should be cleaned and thoroughly aseptisized, especially where there is soilage from a patient. *Preparing and cleaning the OR for the next case is routinely performed by an orderly designated specifically for this job.*

Chapter 10
Setting Up Your OR Suite

Scrubbing

Of course, it is expected that you will perform a proper scrubbing of your hands and arms. Depending on your ASC's protocols, there will be water and brush scrubs or perhaps alcohol-based scrubs. For the first scrub of the day, we suggest a full soap-based scrubbing of hands and arms with under-nail cleaning usually supplied in self-contained scrub systems with sponge, liquid soap/antiseptic. Subsequent scrubs using waterless alcohol-based systems have become popular and seem to be adequate for asepsis. Follow the manufacturer's directions.

Be sure that all non-sterile needs are addressed prior to scrubbing. Once scrubbed, all non-sterile requirements will be handled by your circulator – these are personnel who can assist in non-sterile tasks such as retrieving additional instruments, adjusting the microscope, and positioning the patient. Be aware that once scrubbed, the space below your waist and behind you is not considered sterile so that your hands should always be placed in front and above the waist (Fig. 10.1).

Before initiating surgery, you should perform a "site check" of your surroundings, assuring yourself that all systems are go. There should be available within your sight line a legible list of tools and habits associated with your surgeon. This is usually hung on the wall near your table (see Appendix A).

Anesthesia

Your surgeon, in conjunction with the anesthesiologist – and pre-clearance notes and admonitions supplied by the patient's primary care physician, if included – will make the determination as to what type of anesthesia should be used in each case. Considerations might depend on the patient's age and state of health, prescribed medications, anxiety level, and the anticipated complexity of the surgery. Patients

© Springer Nature Switzerland AG 2020
R. S. Koplin et al., *The Scrub's Bible*,
https://doi.org/10.1007/978-3-030-44345-0_10

Fig. 10.1 Super Scrub
reminds you to maintain
sterile posture
once gowned

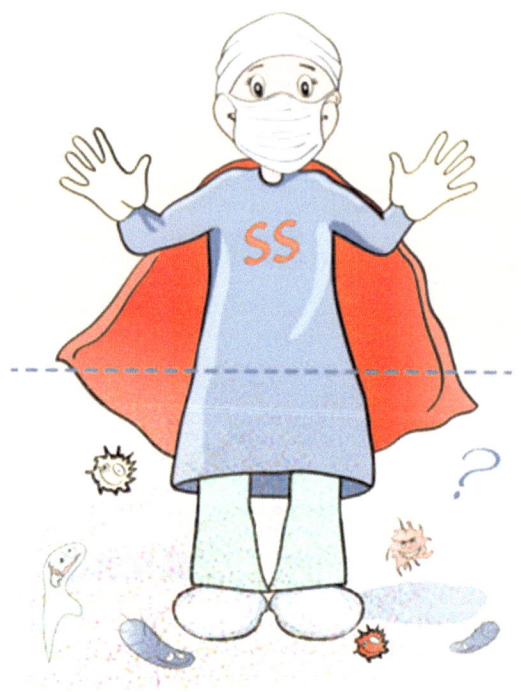

who have their cataract surgeries performed at an ASC generally have been prese-lected for either topical or a regional anesthetic block under monitored anesthesia care (MAC).

Local anesthesia, injected xylocaine commonly, provides numbness to the local-ized area where the anesthetic is delivered. In the case of modern cataract surgery topical anesthesia – eye drops are popular. Eye drops that may be utilized include 0.5% tetracaine and 0.5% proparacaine. The patient is usually dosed in the preop-erative holding area, and this will usually be supplemented once the patient is in the OR. 1% lidocaine may also be used by some surgeons in a gel form.

Because topical anesthetics provide numbness only to the surface of the eye, manipulation of structures within the eye (such as the iris) may still cause some patient discomfort if touched by surgical instruments. For this reason, many sur-geons will supplement topical anesthesia with an injection of anesthetic into the eye once the surgery starts. Intracameral, non-preserved 1% lidocaine, when injected in modest amounts into the anterior chamber, is generally safe and effective. Anesthetics containing preservatives can be toxic to the corneal endothelium and to the retina and are to be avoided.

In some instances, your surgeon may elect to use regional anesthesia which pro-vides more a comprehensive anesthesia to the anatomy, including the lids and skin around the eye, as well as akinesia (arrests muscle movement) to the extraocular muscles for a relatively prolonged period. Corneal transplant surgeons typically use a peribulbar block (anesthetic injection into the orbit) since there may be manipulation of sensitive anatomy in the eye.

Peribulbar anesthetic is particularly helpful if a patient is unusually anxious and exhibits a low threshold for manipulation, or if the surgery is anticipated to be lengthier, or if immobilizing eye movement is advantageous. Besides a peribulbar injection, an injection may be given either beneath the conjunctiva (rarely) or deeper into the orbit (a retrobulbar injection).

Because retrobulbar anesthesia is administered deep into the orbit where there are delicate structures such as the eye itself, the optic nerve, extraocular muscles, and blood vessels, retrobulbar anesthesia can in, rare cases, cause complications. Among these are perforations of the eye with the needle and the potential of irreversible vision loss, permanent double vision if muscle damage occurs, cardiorespiratory arrest, or an orbital hemorrhage if a blood vessel is inadvertently damaged. In some procedures, a peribulbar block is preferred over retrobulbar block because of the lower risk of local and systemic complications. In addition to topical/regional anesthesia, most cataract surgery at ASCs is performed under monitored anesthesia care (MAC). This requires the presence of an anesthesiologist (MD) or, alternatively, a nurse anesthetist working under the direction of an anesthesiologist.

In most cases an IV is inserted, usually in the anticubital fossa (where the elbow bends) or the back of the hand or forearm. This allows the anesthesiologist to keep the patient hydrated and is the vehicle for the delivery of required drugs such as soporifics (makes the patient drowsy) and analgesics (diminishes pain sensation) or corticosteroids for inflammation. Agents commonly used include short-acting opioid analgesic such as a fentanyl derivative, a benzodiazepine such as midazolam, or a sedative like propofol. Midazolam and propofol have the additional effect of causing amnesia so that the patient may not remember the procedure. These agents are generally extremely safe in the dosages given for cataract surgery, though fentanyl can cause nausea, dry mouth, confusion, and weakness and propofol is associated with low blood pressure and transient apnea (suspension of breathing).

Patient Prep

The prepping process begins in earnest once an orderly has assisted the patient to the OR suite. A circulator will then begin preparing the patient for the sterile procedure. The OR tech or circulator will assist the patient onto the operating table and will ensure that the patient is in a comfortable supine position (facing up). The circulator will provide blankets and cushions as needed. Once comfortably ensconced on the operating table, the patient should be reassured that all is well and reminded that once the prep begins, they should not move their head, arms, or feet. Making sure that patient finds a comfortable place of rest for all three will reduce the likelihood that they will move during surgery. The patient should be admonished not to touch their face once prepped. If the patient appears to be moving their legs in spite of admonitions, they may have a condition called "restless leg syndrome." If this is suspected, the anesthesiologist should be alerted prior to draping the patient for surgery.

The circulator and scrub should make sure that the patient's head is placed so that it is level, neither chin up or chin down. Either situation may put the lids in conflict with adequate visualization of the eye, and the lids may be covering a good portion of the cornea and make surgery difficult. Once you are assured that the patient is in an appropriate position, the circulator will place a drop or two of topical anesthetic – or at the surgeon's preference – lidocaine gel (in belief that it is longer acting) usually in both eyes. (Placing the anesthetic in both eyes is necessary since the urge to blink one eye will automatically blink the fellow eye.)

Blood pressure and EKG are the main functional parameters measured as surgery is initiated along with pulse rate, oxygen saturation, and body temperature. Once in the OR, an oximeter will be affixed to the patient's finger. The patient's blood oxygen saturation is a good reflection of efficient respiration and helps the anesthesiologist monitor the effect of any drug that might depress respirations.

Modern blood pressure systems are automated but annoying to the patient as they feel the cuff tense tightly against their arm every 4–5 minutes. It is best to alert the patient to this process prior to surgery. The EKG machine is generally silent unless an abnormality is encountered or a lead falls away.

Figure 10.2 shows a pulse ox/EKG/BP cuff.

Generally, an IV is inserted in the preoperative area; if not, it will certainly be done immediately on entering the OR suite. If a peribulbar or retrobulbar anesthetic is to be used, the injection will be delivered either by the anesthesiologist or by the surgeon (once a short-acting sedative is provided the patient via the IV). Occasionally this may be given in the preoperative area.

To prepare for a peribulbar or retrobulbar block, ask the circulator for a 5 or 10 cc syringe and a 25 gauge needle. After wiping the elastic covering to the medication vial with an alcohol swipe, you will withdraw the proscribed amount from the vial (typically a mixture of Xylocaine and Marcaine and often with hyaluronidase to increase tissue penetration). If this is being prepared *after* scrubbing, the vial will be held for you by the circulator. You will exchange needles, placing either a short 25 gauge needle (peribulbar injection) or a long 25 gauge needle or a specially designed blunted retrobulbar needle (retrobulbar injection) on the syringe to be used by your surgeon to deliver the drug. This syringe – and any other on your tray – should be clearly identified with a prepared identification sticker (a package of "sticky" identification labels should be attached to the various syringe on your table) (Fig. 10.3).

A standard antiseptic scrub is then performed, often by the circulator wearing sterile gloves. This prep entails using a 10% povidone-iodine scrub over the upper face with both eyes closed. This includes the face, usually above the mid-nose, on the side of the eye being operated on. Then with the lids lifted, the operative eye is carefully washed with 5% povidone-iodine followed by sterile saline, often with a bulb syringe.

Although under most circumstance it would have been evaluated in the pre-op area, it is good form to check the dilation of the pupil prior to the surgeon taking

Fig. 10.2 Pulse ox/EKG/
BP cuff. (Photographer:
Bob Masini)

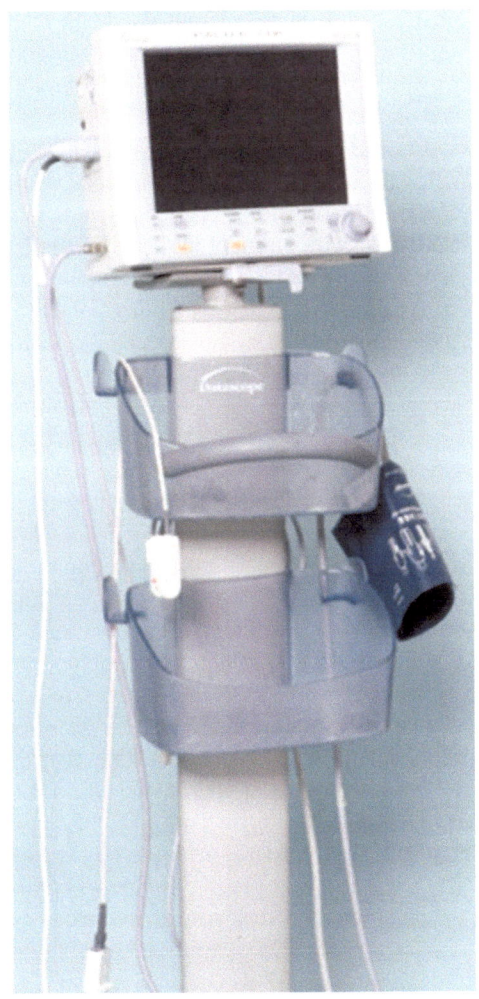

Fig. 10.3 Anesthetic.
(Photographer:
Bob Masini)

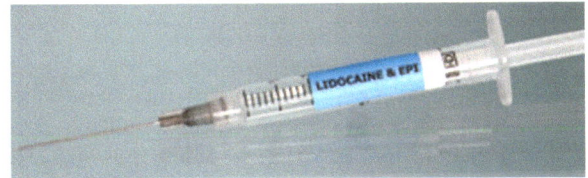

their seat. The degree of dilation should be reported to the surgeon. A well-dilated
pupil – say 7–10 mm – is ideal, while pupils that are around 5 mm, or less, might
suggest that attention is required. Partially dilated pupils may be caused by pseudo-
exfoliation, a condition often associated with loose zonules, or certain drugs such as
Flomax (used mainly for enlarged prostate conditions) or other alpha-blocking

pharmaceuticals. Poor pupillary dilation may also be associated with previous eye surgery, trauma, or inflammatory disease of the front of the eye. Reminding your surgeon of the status of the pupil is not only appropriate but signals that you are alert and partnered with them.

Prior to draping the patient – and in the presence of the operating surgeon – you will call for a "time out," where final confirmation is made of the patient's name, date of birth, eye to be operated (where the surgeon has marked the eye to be operated upon with an indelible fat pen; the letters should be at least partially visible once draped), and the lens implant power and model to be used, as well as the date of expiration. The surgeon is then asked to confirm these facts. The unopened box containing the IOL is shown to the surgeon for confirmation using a primary source (e.g., the calculations in the surgeon's record). A verbal response from the surgeon is required. Grunting is not an acceptable response.

A surgeon's greatest respect is reserved for scrubs and technicians who consistently pay attention to details and exhibit a determined sense of anticipation in the OR. This suggests to the surgeon that his or her team is fully invested in the procedure – always aware of their surroundings – are not daydreaming or seemingly bored. This sense of dedication to the procedure at hand provides great confidence to the surgeon.

Scrubs alert to the ongoing surgical procedure are more aware of the needs of their surgeon and understand the surgeon's temperament, style of surgery, and instrument needs (and yes their peculiar idiosyncrasies: oh, did we really say that?). Indeed, a great scrub seems, at times, to be able to read their surgeon's mind. Often there is a close bond and respect forged – sometimes unstated but certainly mutually appreciated – between surgeon and scrub.

For each patient brought to the OR, it is typical that an 8 × 11 sheet of paper with pertinent patient information – identifying the patent's name, surgical eye, and perhaps lens power, printed in large type – be placed in a conspicuous place (see Appendix B). So, as you can see, the personnel at your ASC go to extensive lengths to avoid operating on the wrong patient, the wrong eye, or using a misidentified lens implant.

Draping

Finally, and only after confirming all the above, the patient is covered with a sterile drape (usually of a treated paper material, less likely a cloth gown) that covers all but the eye to be operated and usually extends to the knees or beyond (measuring about 4 feet in width and 5–6 feet in length).

Occasionally a patient will express concerns about claustrophobia, and a technique which elevates the bottom of the drape, taping it high above the operating table to some extension device, will give the patient a sense of openness that will make them feel more comfortable. The anesthesiologist will have the option of providing oxygen to the patient's nose.

The patient should be reminded to keep their head still, eyes up to the operating scope light (apologizing for the brightness but reassuring them that this will tend to fade in a few minutes) and admonishing them not to move their arms or legs.

Once draped, it is helpful if you speak to the patient in a soothing and empathetic voice and inform the patient that if there is something causing distress, or if they feel a cough or sneeze developing, they can quietly – without undue body movement – inform the surgeon or scrub of their concern.

Most ASCs use disposable plastic lid drapes to cover the upper and lower lids. This sequesters the eyelashes under plastic and helps avoid a potential source of contamination. These drapes are usually a strip of soft plastic with backing provided in the "pak" (sometimes supplied as one for each eye, or occasionally one large drape to be cut in two). You will strip the backing away and hand the sticky piece face down to the surgeon trying to avoid getting it tangled on the surgeon's glove. Alternatively, your surgeon may expect you to place the drapes for them. To do so, you must "capture" the lashes and lay them against the lid just at the margins, pressing the drape down against the forehead in the case of the upper lid and then again on the lower lid against the cheek. This may take some practice.

Alternatively, your ASC will provide a Steri-Drape© (Fig. 10.4) that is smaller and easier to use but must be cut in half. The most efficient way to hand the drape to your surgeon is to direct the partially peeled (from the paper backing) sections to your surgeon and allow them to peel it completely away. This way the surgeon does not have to guess which side is sticky.

The eye is held open for the surgery using a small speculum (Fig. 10.5) which is generally made of stainless steel or titanium. There are screw type speculums, allowing the surgeon to set the degree of spacing, and wire speculums that are

Fig. 10.4 Steri-Drapes. (Photographer: Bob Masini)

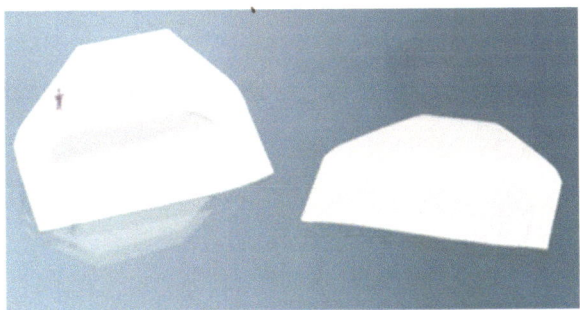

Fig. 10.5 Speculum (our stock image)

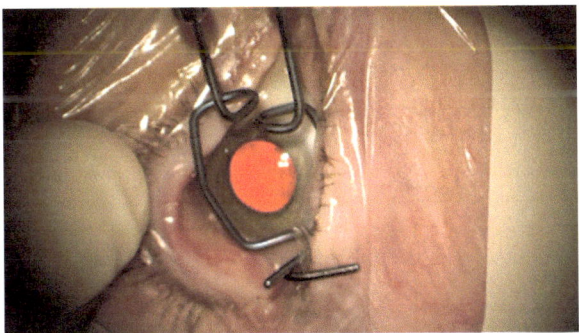

spring-like and are one size fits all. Some of these are oriented so that they are placed open to the temporal side (toward the ear), while others open on the nasal side (over the bridge of the nose).

Instrumentation

There are certain instruments that are universal to the procedure known as phaco-emulsification. Then there are instruments and devices that are peculiar to specific surgeons and their techniques.

Many of the handheld instruments on your tray are delicate and expensive and require care and respect, or they will be wasted or in need of costly repair. Other instruments are no less valuable from a technical point of view but are either disposable or used two or three times. We will attempt to cover the most common variations.

Basic Instrument Table

Once surgery has begun, your instrument table is your domain and you are to control its environment (Fig. 10.6). You are to protect and defend it. It is up to you to make sure that the table is populated with all the instruments and supporting paraphernalia for that particular surgeon and for the type of cataract operation being considered.

Be prepared for curve balls. Occasionally your surgeon will intend to perform a routine phacoemulsification procedure, but then finds that there is an extenuating circumstance forcing a change in plans. Your surgeon might, in spite of having initiated a phacoemulsification procedure, announce that they intend, instead, to perform an ECCE (extracapsular cataract extraction) or ICCE (intracapsular cataract extraction). This is described as a "conversion."

Your instrument table should be set for the most common challenges, and, as well, you should know where in the OR suite all of the other required instruments are stored.

Please review the section defined as The Surgical Tray. It will describe the multiple instruments and additional materials required to initiate and support variations in cataract procedures.

How to Hand Instruments to Your Surgeon

All instruments are handed to the surgeon with the handle side toward them (Fig. 10.7). Likewise, your surgeon should hand them back in similar fashion.

Fig. 10.6 Super Scrub
defending instrument table

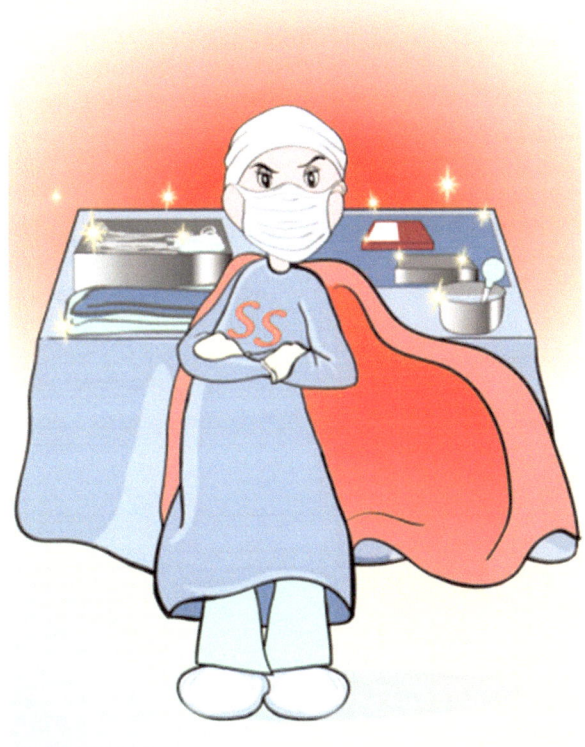

Fig. 10.7 Handing
instruments.
(Photographer:
Bob Masini)

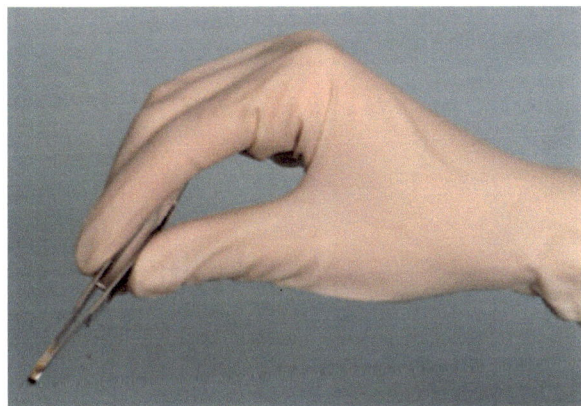

It is your job to have the desired instrument reach the surgeon comfortably (they should not have to stretch to reach your hand), and at times they will simply place their hand out – palm side up – in expectation that you will gently, but firmly, place the instrument handle fully in their hand. An instrument should be placed with moderate but sincere force, and you should let go only when you understand that the surgeon has completely grasped the instrument.

After a few experiences with your surgeon, you should know in which hand a surgeon expects an instrument to be placed. Although it is true that most surgeons prefer one hand over the other when retrieving an instrument, you will occasionally be surprised to find a surgeon confuse you with an unexpected preference. This is more common in naturally left-handed surgeons who have learned to use their right hand for certain chores.

You'll know that you have reached the Zen level of surgical scrubbing when, without a word passing between the two of you, your surgeon simply puts their hand out and you understand with confidence which instrument they are expecting.

No one is perfect. If your surgeon tends to occasionally return instruments to you with the sharp or operating side of the device toward you, you should remind them to turn the instrument before advancing it toward you. You should not, however, do this at the time of surgery, while the patient might be aware of such interactions. It will diminish the surgeon in the patient's eyes; a decided No-No.

Chapter 11
The Phaco Machine

There are several phaco machines on the American market. Conceptually they are all tasked with accomplishing the same outcome: a safe and efficient phacoemulsification of the human lens. Each device is marketed with various features and benefits that may or may not work to your surgeon's advantage. Your surgeon will find a comfort level with one system or another although many centers offer only a single system due to expense, training, and the challenge of maintaining inventory.

Understanding a modicum of the innards of the phaco machine – which we will present in a relatively nontechnical manner – is indispensable. No, you are not expected to solve all the problems associated with these sophisticated systems; however, you will be surprised at how adept at troubleshooting a device you can become with a bit of experience.

The Components

The standard phaco machine will incorporate the following:

Console This is the body of the phaco machine (Fig. 11.1). The console, set on rollers, houses the software modules, video monitor and controls, pumps, connection for cassette functions including aspiration and infusion tubing, and electronics used to drive the system.

Display A touch screen that displays the settings, elemental data accumulation (such as length of surgery, power applications, etc.), and surgeon performance is placed front and center on the console. Surgeon settings are usually pre-programmed and are resident in the menu (noted as surgeon "preferences"). Changes in surgeon settings including fluid aspiration, vacuum, power, and fluid infusion can be made on the fly as the surgeon confronts challenges to the surgery (more on this later).

© Springer Nature Switzerland AG 2020
R. S. Koplin et al., *The Scrub's Bible*,
https://doi.org/10.1007/978-3-030-44345-0_11

Fig. 11.1 Console. (Photographer: Bob Masini)

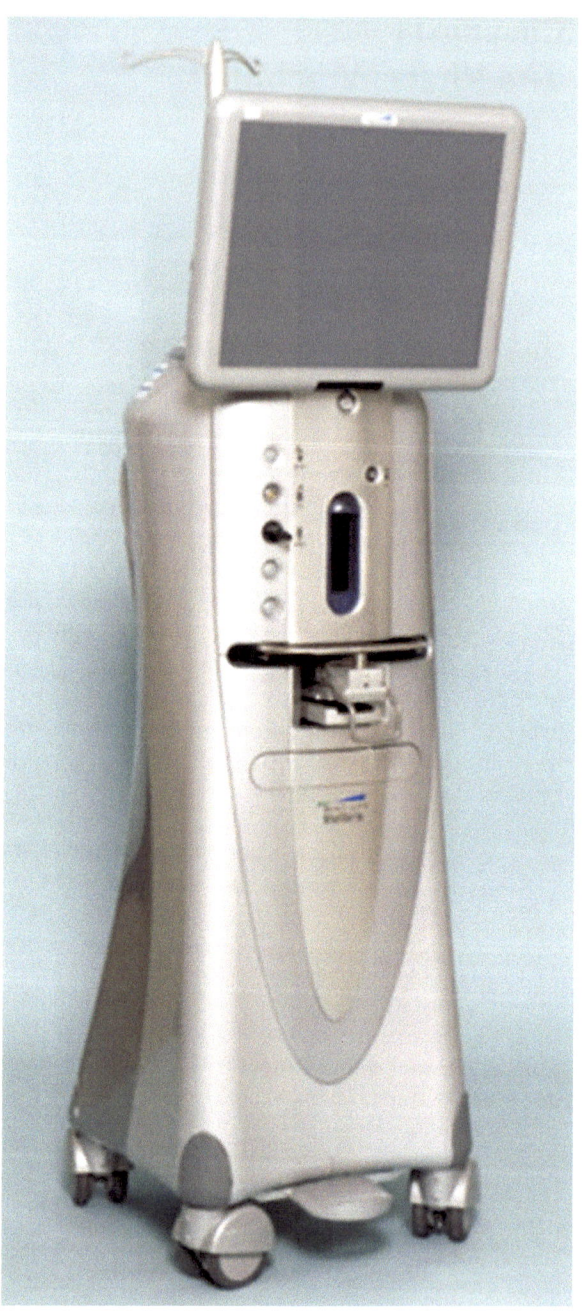

Phaco Handpiece: Needle and Sleeve The handpiece is the heart of the operative end of the phaco system and contains a device known to engineers as "horn." The horn contains a unique crystal (piezo) that when stimulated by an electrical current vibrates and in turn drives a hollow, metallic needle (often titanium) to ultrasonic frequencies, resulting in a powerfully vibrating tool.

The hollow needle at the operating end of the handpiece is ensconced in a flexible silicone sleeve, and infusion fluid is delivered between the sleeve and the needle to exit the sleeve via two exits (ports) at its far end. At the butt end of the handpiece are two fittings which will be attached to tubing's from the console. As previously noted, but worth repeating, one is for the fluid infusion (fluids going in the eye) and the other where the emulsified lens material will exit from the eye (aspiration). The lens waste – now in a fluid mix – is deposited in a plastic receptacle attached to the phaco console.

The business section of the handpiece – the hollow titanium needle measuring 7–9 mm in length and screwed to the shaft – is driven to an ultrasonic frequency, and its resultant motion can be directed back and forth like a jackhammer (called longitudinal) or oscillatory, or a combination of motions, in order to fragment/emulsify (break up) the nucleus of the lens. The needle may be straight or curved (30° or 45°). Angulated needles tend to deliver more power.

The phaco needle comes packaged along with silicone sleeves which are screwed to the handpiece and are tightened using a small "wrench" of sorts which is supplied with the manufacturer's kit. The silicone sleeve is threaded over the needle tip to the shaft. There are two openings (ports) located at the very far end of the silicone sleeve 180 degrees apart. Fluid infusion into the eye is provided through these ports afforded by the space between the sleeve and the phaco needle. An important secondary gain is the cooling effect of the infusion fluid running along the shaft of the heat generating (vibrating) phaco needle. Without this process serious corneal burns are likely.

The phaco needle's hollow shaft serves as a conduit for the emulsified nuclear material aspirated from the anterior chamber along with infusion fluids to a disposal unit (cassette) hanging on the console.

Bimanual Handpieces (Fig. 11.2) These may or may not be supplied with your phaco machine. If available, your surgeon may choose to split the two functions of the single handpiece (known as coaxial surgery and includes infusion and aspiration) and instead use two separate tools – one handpiece for ultrasound/aspiration and the other purely for infusion of fluid. Similar split functions are available for the IA process as well. Surgeons may opt for this if they wish to operate through rather small openings (as small as 1.2–1.5 mm compared to 2.2 mm, 2.7 mm, or 3.0 mm).

Figure 11.3 shows a Phaco needle protruding beyond the silicone sleeve.

Irrigation and Aspiration (I&A or IA) Handpiece It is a pencil-thin metal device with infusion and aspiration functions but *without* phaco capability, used to remove soft cortical and epinuclear material and viscoelastic after phacoemulsification of the nucleus. Like phaco tips, I&A tips can be straight or curved (45, 90, or 180

Fig. 11.2 Phaco
handpiece. (Photographer:
Bob Masini)

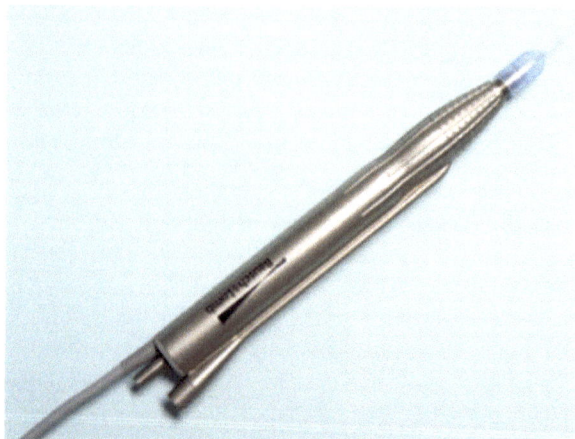

Fig. 11.3 Phaco needle
protruding beyond silicone
sleeve (Koplin stock)

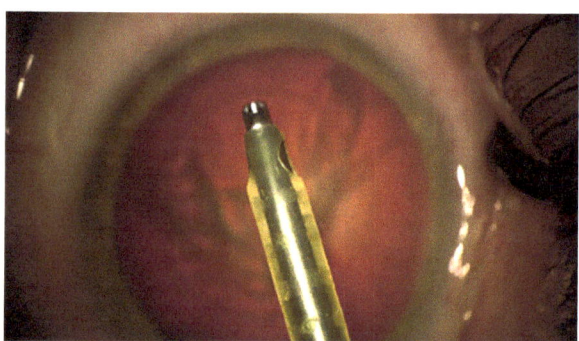

degrees). Curved I&A handpieces are helpful in removing material directly under
the surgeon's main entry wound into the eye.

Tubings Clear plastic tubes are provided for both infusions into the AC from a bag
or bottle of "normal" saline and a second tubing provided to service the aspiration
of fluid and lens materials from the AC into a bag hanging from the phaco console.
The two tubes (the infusion tube is thicker than the aspiration tube) are inserted at
the back end of the phaco handpiece (as well as the I&A handpiece when in use).
Since the connections for the infusion and aspiration lines on the various handpieces
are sized and shaped differently, it is virtually impossible to place the two tubes onto
the wrong instrument receptacle.

Cassette This disposable mechanism is included in the "phaco pack." The cassette
generally will be fitted into a receptacle at the side or back of the phaco console. The
cassette receives the contents of the aspiration tubing, collecting emulsified lens
material and fluid aspirate.

Pump This generates movement of fluid along the aspiration line so that the emulsified lens material will be drawn out of the eye and into a cassette attached to the phaco

console. Phaco machines on the market comprise of either the peristaltic pump (flow based), venturi pump (vacuum based), or a hybrid. These functions are strictly of concern to the surgeon; however, you may be asked to alter basic settings on the console. In newer generations of systems, sensor-controlled infusion has been introduced.

Remote Console Controls Along with a touch screen display, your phaco system will be provided with a remote control device which is tucked into a sterile sleeve typically found with the phaco-pak. Once in the sterile sleeve, the remote will sit on an arm that slides from the console that will likewise be covered with a sterile plastic drape. The sterile drape allows you to place the handpiece and other sterile devices securely on the stand. The remote control device allows you (or the circulator if you prefer) to adjust functions without leaning over to touch the console.

Surgical Foot pedal A multipurpose foot pedal is either wired or blue toothed to the console. The foot pedal performs some of the functions duplicated on the console, while other functions can only be controlled from the foot pedal. The foot pedal is to be placed under the foot preferred by your surgeon. (During the setup process, make sure the circulator changes the positioning of the microscope and phaco foot pedals as required, depending on which side of the table your surgeon will be sitting.)

In the phaco mode, the foot pedal provides several functions including infusion, or infusion with aspiration, or infusion, aspiration, and ultrasound-phaco simultaneously. Kicking the foot pedal to the left will cause reverse flow from the infusion port. (If your surgeon has accidentally captured the capsule during the IA portion of the operation, this reverse or regurgitation mode is handy.)

There are three surgeon modes for phaco: sculpt, segment removal, and epinuclear removal. Each process is specific for events in the eye and pertains almost exclusively to how a surgeon approaches nuclear disassembly (how the nucleus is broken up and removed from the eye). As the surgeon moves the procedure along they will announce which mode they desire. You will simply engage the specific button.

Phaco-pak To function, phaco machines require certain disposable items. Invariably these will be provided by the manufacturer as a "phaco-pak." Packs may be provided with only the basic setup requirements or may be expanded to include just about everything needed to complete a procedure. Your ASC will decide how to customize the pack: i.e., what is included in a pack and what will be purchased independently.

An example of this might be a bundled product containing most, if not all, of the disposables associated with the phacoemulsification machine along with drapes, phaco tips, sleeves, and tubing, as well as the blades and many of the fluids, drugs, syringes, cannulas, identification labels, and viscoelastics required to complete the procedure. The bundled pack system is not only helpful to the inventory process, but there is often a cost savings as well. The phaco-pak (Fig. 11.4) is also helpful to the scrub nurse since most of the required elements needed for surgery are sitting right there in front of you.

Fig. 11.4 A Phaco cassette
with tubing pack.
(Photographer:
Bob Masini)

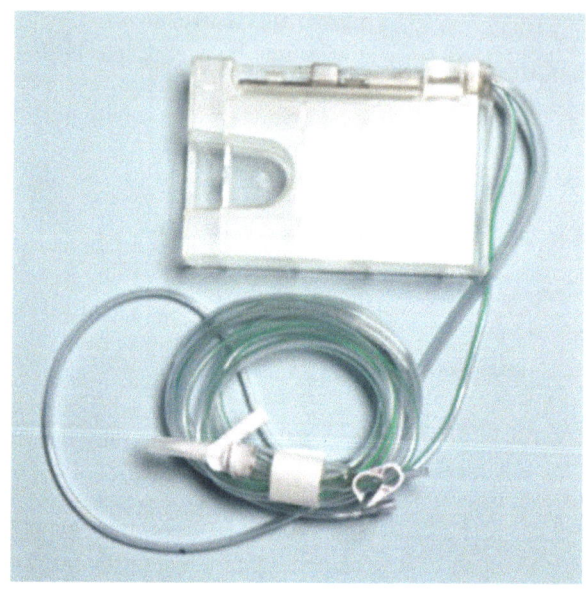

How Fluid Gets in and out of the Eye During Phaco Surgery

Balancing Fluid Infusion with Aspiration: Maintaining a Desirable IOP

A. Standard Gravity-Fed Infusion Infusion fluid (also called balanced saline fluid) entering the eye through one of the two plastic tubes attached to the phaco handpiece (one infusion the other aspiration) is then attached to an IV bottle or fluid-filled plastic bag which itself is then attached to an IV stand or adjustable rod attached to the phaco console.

The rod can be raised or lowered mechanically. The infusion tubing (usually this is the larger diameter tubing) runs from the bottle to the handpiece delivering infusion fluid via gravity into the anterior chamber, preventing it from collapsing during surgery and mixing with the phaco emulsate to make a soupy mixture of lens and saline that is aspirated from the eye.

The rod may be elevated or lowered by engaging the appropriate button on a remote control or from the menu screen on the console. When the anterior chamber requires greater depth, the bottle may be moved higher. In cases where the eye is very large and there is a tendency for the fluid pressure to press the lens back deeper in the eye, it may be advantageous to lower the bottle height. Your surgeon will signal you to needed changes in the bottle height based on how well the anterior chamber of the eye is behaving during the phaco procedure.

In very prolonged cases, the bottle or bag may need replacement with a full complement of saline. However, newer consoles may have sensing devices that

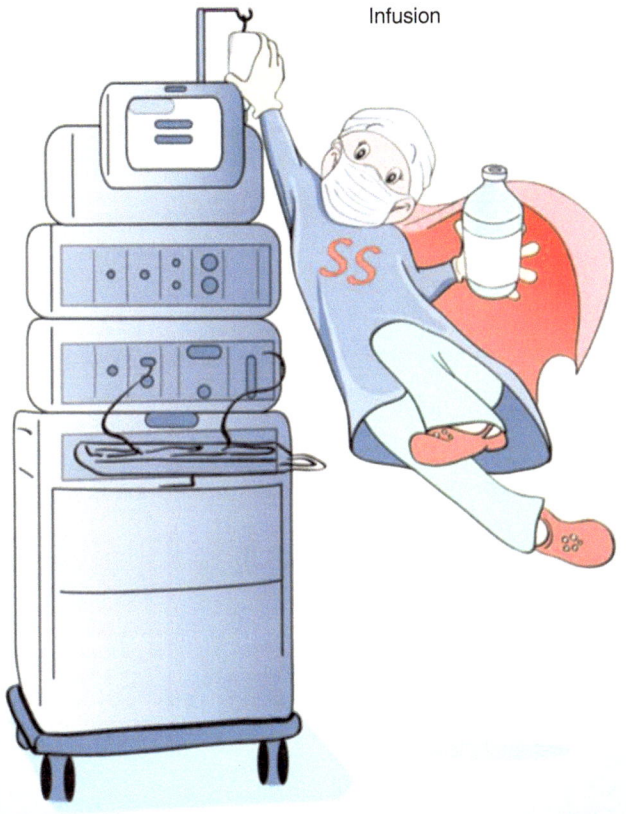

Fig. 11.5 Super Scrub whisking empty bottle (infusion), and replacing it with a full bottle

announce that there is a need to replace the bottle. The lack of normal infusion volume may lead to a sudden collapse of the anterior chamber, and if the surgeon is unaware and has instruments in the eye, there is risk of damage to the cornea, iris, lens, or its capsule. Well in advance of the need, announce to your surgeon that the infusion bottle must be changed. In the interim the surgeon will remove all instruments from the eye (Fig. 11.5).

B. Pump/Sensor-Controlled Infusion If your ASC has recently purchased new phaco machines, it is likely that the infusion is performed by a pump mechanism massaging and plastic bag placed within the console itself. Sensors placed in proximity to the tubing described by the aspiration-infusion loop actively monitor the IOP and attempt to maintain the set point defined by your surgeon prior to surgery.

Chapter 12
Setting up the Phaco Machine

Each phaco system has its own "setup" procedures and they are generally quite user-friendly since the entire process is menu driven directly from the console screen.

Since modern phaco consoles are digital, once powered up the systems will go through a "booting" phase, initializing the system, just like any PC. This will be followed by a series of system tests verifying the various machine functions. Finally, there will be a priming process which will test the adequacy of the pump and tubing and finally a tuning process that will test the ultrasonic handpiece. You will be required to respond to screen directions at appropriate times during the priming and tuning process, so pay attention. However, the entire process takes only minutes.

Generic Menu Options

Regardless of which phaco machine your surgeon uses, all console screens detailing system functions will have similar controls even if they are called something different (Fig. 12.1).

There are four basic phaco machine settings important for surgery (although there are additions to this based on the manufacturer's features, such as pump sensor infusion setting to avoid unusual deepening of the anterior chamber in highly near-sighted eyes).

Power settings This reflects the power at the tip of the phaco handpiece – the phaco needle – which translates to longitudinal movement of the tip (think of the tip pounding the nucleus in a forward and back motion) and associated fragmentation by ultrasound. As an important aside, the higher the power, the more heat produced, and we will discuss this further on. Once the parameters are set, they are controlled by the surgeon using the foot pedal. The foot pedal in this case functions like an accelerator; the deeper it is depressed the higher the modes rise to preset maximums.

© Springer Nature Switzerland AG 2020
R. S. Koplin et al., *The Scrub's Bible*,
https://doi.org/10.1007/978-3-030-44345-0_12

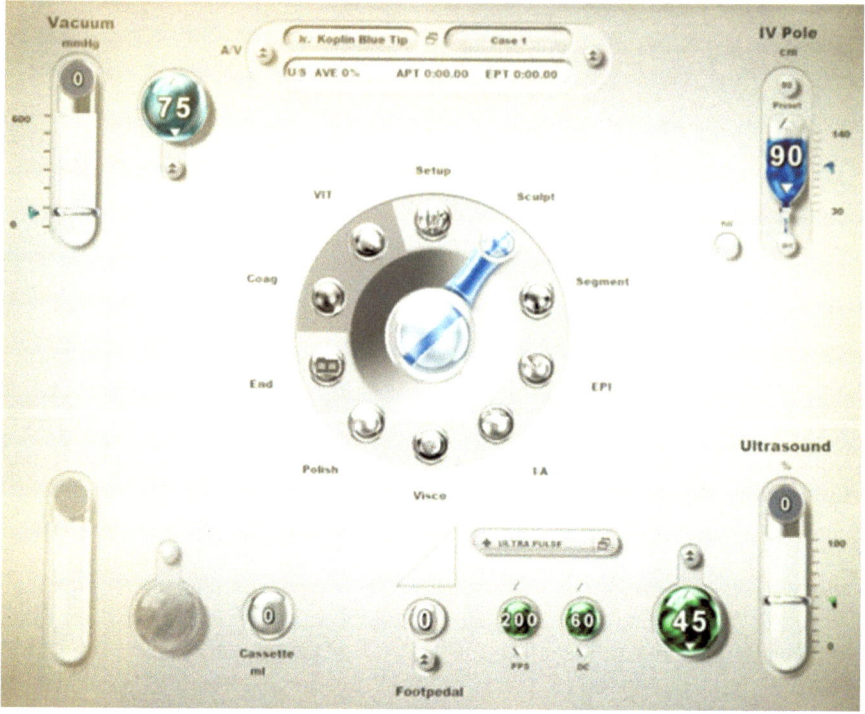

Fig. 12.1 Close-up of menu screen. (Photographer: Bob Masini)

Power settings typically go from 0% to 100% as a reflection of percent of available preset power. If the phaco machine includes an oscillatory or lateral sweeping component as well (meaning the tip also has rotational or lateral movement in addition to longitudinal movement), there will be settings for these as well.

Vacuum settings   These will typically be set between 0 and 400 mmHg. Vacuum is a function that is best described by what happens when the port (or opening at the tip) is occluded. Consider a vacuum cleaner when you place your palm over its opening. A rapid suction develops keeping your hand tightly adhered to the opening. This is a good thing when using the phaco portion of the system: think of holding the back of the head of a boxing opponent while you pummel them. Not very fair, but very efficient. So, the goal is to keep the nuclear fragment on the tip while it is being pounded. (A note about this: heat is generated during this process. The surgeon should avoid crimping the infusion line – which acts a coolant – since decreasing or stopping the flow of fluid results in an immediate buildup of heat. This may cause a serious burn to corneal tissue.)

In sculpting mode vacuum is usually set to a low value. Once nuclear segments are prepared (freely mobile) for removal, the system is placed in quadrant removal mode, and here vacuum is raised to a level comfortable to the surgeon's technique which can be as high as 400 mmHg.

Aspiration Flow Rate Settings Aspiration represents the amount of fluid passing through the port during a defined period, typically labeled in cc per minute.

Your surgeon will have had experience at various settings and will request changes depending on the recalcitrant nature of the lens material being addressed in both the phaco and IA modes.

A note about aspiration and vacuum settings: high settings tend to invite sudden surges in fluid when the vacuum is broken, and the tissue occluding the port may be aspirated with startling suddenness. This could threaten the integrity of the capsule. (Unusually high settings in all phaco functions are something left to very experienced and intrepid surgeons.)

Bottle height The bottle height on the rod-stand is automatically adjusted when your surgeon switches functions. The bottle height (typically 70–110 cm above eye level) controls how much infusion fluid goes into the eye (higher bottle more flow). The bottle height is usually a preset function but can be manually overridden if your surgeon desires a change in bottle height.

Personal surgeon settings Most phaco systems have within their computer functions files capable of storing surgeon-specific personalized settings for each stage of the surgery, thus eliminating the need to change settings unless asked to do so by the surgeon.

Once the system has booted, go to the screen icon for Personalized Settings, open the file folder, and choose the name of the surgeon or add a surgeon and choose the basic settings to install. As your surgeon progress through each stage of the surgery, you will be asked to advance to the settings of the next stage. Occasionally, your surgeon will ask to change a setting that may have been previously preset. Outside of the surgeon's profile settings all console settings and resets during active surgery will no influence preference settings. It is good practice to announce to your surgeon whenever you have made the requested change (i.e., "Bottle height increased to 90," "Phaco power to 65").

Chapter 13
Troubleshooting the Phaco Machine

Being capable of trouble shooting the system is very important. When the system set up goes smoothly, it's intuitive, takes only a few minutes, and requires very little additional input from you. But when the system comes back with a balky message suggesting that something is amiss, this is where you earn the big bucks.

Surgeons tend to get very impatient with troubled devices, and not uncommonly they are not that familiar enough with the systems themselves to be able to assist you in solving the problem. So, often when there is a breakdown in the OR, the harsh light of expectancy will be shinning on you. Some examples:

Has the system booted but will not access functions?

- Close down the system and reboot.
- Take the plug out and leave it out for 30 seconds to a minute.
- Call the manufacturer's Help Line.

Is there fluid running down the handpiece?

- Is the tubing tightly in place around all connections?
- Tubes are mostly attached via "friction" connection. Sometimes these may be wet and easily slide out of place. Reconnect with vigor.

The phaco tip is chattering or there is little or no phaco function:

- Is the tip (needle) securely screwed into place?
- It is not uncommon to fail to tighten the phaco needle completely. Remove the silicone sleeve on the phaco tip and use the block-like wrench to tighten the needle appropriately (but not to the point where it will be a major chore removing it).

Why is the aspiration mal-functioning? (Oddly, the set up and tuning have gone well, but the surgeon notes a failure to aspirate properly.)

© Springer Nature Switzerland AG 2020
R. S. Koplin et al., *The Scrub's Bible*,
https://doi.org/10.1007/978-3-030-44345-0_13

- Is there a blockage in the handpiece (tip or body of the phaco instrument)?

   Use a syringe with saline to forcefully clear the aspiration line in the instrument.

- Is the cassette properly inserted in the console?

Occasionally the cassette will need to be removed from its attachment to the chassis and reconnected. If a message continues to flash on the screen suggesting that the cassette is faulty, it may be one of the tubing lines. In this case it is best to bite the bullet and replace the entire cassette and tubing. (Save the old tubing since if it proves to be the culprit, a refund is owed to the ASC; penny saved is a penny earned.)

Chapter 14
Cataract Surgery: More than One Way to Skin a Cat

Simply stated cataract surgery is the removal of a cloudy, dysfunctional crystalline lens (Fig. 14.1). All cataract operations remove some, or all, of the crystalline lens. Virtually all cataract procedures include replacing the cataractous lens with a new, clear lens called an intraocular lens implant (IOL) and manufactured of some type of solid or foldable plastic/acrylic – or occasionally silicone – of a predetermined power.

Cataract surgery can be performed in one of the several ways. The most common approach, as we discussed earlier, is by phacoemulsification. So, as a scrub, when attending to a cataract operation, phacoemulsification surgery is what you will encounter most of the time. The core procedure requires that the surgeon safely open the anterior capsule of the lens in a controlled manner known as a continuous curvilinear

Fig. 14.1 Dense nuclear cataract

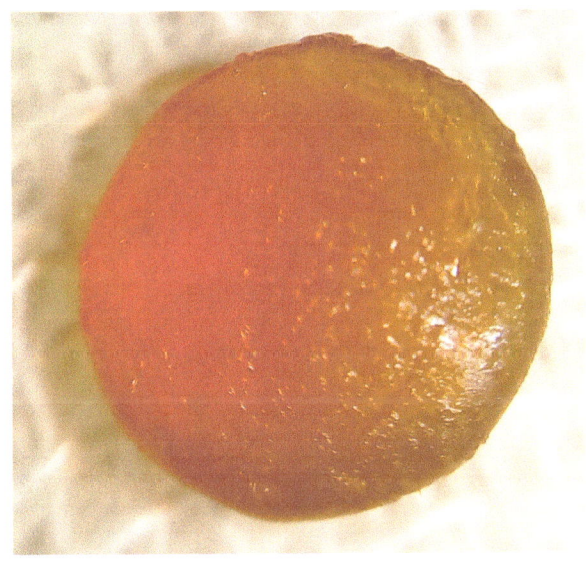

© Springer Nature Switzerland AG 2020
R. S. Koplin et al., *The Scrub's Bible*,
https://doi.org/10.1007/978-3-030-44345-0_14

capsulorrhexis (CCC) to gain access to the cataractous portion of the lens. Done appropriately, this results in an uninterrupted round opening without radial defects which could result in "tear-out" of the capsule to the far periphery and possibly result in lens material being lost posteriorly into the vitreous cavity. (See Femto Laser assisted Cataract Surgery – FLACS – for alternatives to this manual form of capsulotomy.) Once the nuclear portion of the lens (cataract) is laid bare the phacoemulsification process can be initiated.

However, for reasons that may have to do with the hardness of the lens or the weakness of the zonules (and there may be other reasons), your surgeon may opt to perform a planned extracapsular cataract extraction (ECCE) – of which there are several variations. In most cases – except a pars plana vitrectomy-lensectomy technique – an ECCE consists of removing the nucleus of the lens manually, usually in one piece, always intent on leaving the posterior capsule intact.

If a cataractous lens appears incapable of being salvaged through phaco or a form of ECC), and with the potential for the cataractous lens to dislocate into the back of the eye a procedure that consists of the *complete* removal of the lens – with capsule intact and stripped of its remaining zonules – may be the prudent option. This is known as an intracapsular cataract extraction (ICCE).

Classic Extracapsular Cataract Extraction (Fig. 14.2) A classic ECCE will likely be performed utilizing a corneal wound that may be larger by 1–3 mm than the length of a standard phaco wound. In countries where phaco is too expensive to employ, techniques for forcing the nuclear portion of the lens through a relatively small corneal opening are common. This is known as Manual Small Incision Cataract Surgery or MSICS or SICS. Where it performed regulary, the results are quire good, but it is not without its challenges since a very large caapsulotomy is required and there is a fair amount of manipulation of the nucleus to free it from the capsule in order to prepare it for exit from the anterior chamber.) In the classic form of ECCE the nuclear portion of the lens is removed using one of the several techniques for *expressing* the nucleus from the eye. A typical nuclear expression from the capsular bag into the AC would usually include two instruments: one to press on the inferior lip if the wound and a second – such as a small spoonlike device –

Fig. 14.2 Etracapsular cataract extraction

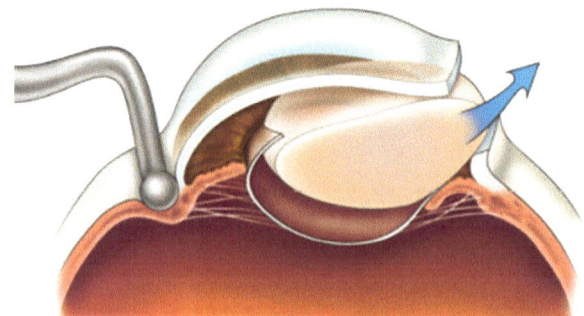

placed over the proximal iris and then slipped beneath the lens. The combination tends to give impetus for the lens to escape through the surgical wound and out of the eye. The corneal wound may then be partially sutured with 10-0 nylon sutures to provide a relatively closed environment and a platform for the irrigation and aspiration (I&A) of the remaining lens remnants (cortical). The IOL is then inserted – either in the remaining capsular bag or above the capsule in the ciliary sulcus (the area just in behind the peripheral iris). At the conclusion of the procedure, depending on the length of the corneal incision and its competency against easy leakage, the remainder of the corneal or scleral wound, may be sutured closed. Multiple sutures might be employed (usually 10-0 nylon).

Variations on Classic Extracapsular Cataract Extraction

Manual Small Incision Extracapsular Cataract Surgery This procedure has found utility especially in regions of the world where the cost of medical care is a major consideration and treating cataracts with high technology – expensive machine and multiple handpieces, along with need to purchase single-use disposable phaco packs and associated materials for each case – is prohibitive.

The procedure itself takes many of the techniques from classic planned ECCE but fits it to a small incision, scleral entry. You should understand that this procedure exists, but it is unlikely that you will be called upon to assist unless you volunteer for a medical mission in a developing country. (There are YouTube videos for your review.)

Pars Plana Approach The pars plana approach is virtually restricted to the realm of a retinal surgeon since there are complexities to be entertained that are generally outside of the skill base of the average anterior segment surgeon. Your surgeon will likely partner with the retinal surgeon to complete this procedure. If the lens is stable enough, the retinal specialist will phaco or use a specialized cutter to remove the lens from behind and within the vitreous cavity. If the cataractous lens can be attacked from behind and the anterior capsule left relatively intact this may result results in a relatively secure scaffold for the implantation of a three-piece IOL secured in the ciliary sulcus. Alternatives in this case, are to place a three piece IOL secured with sutures – or glue – or sutured to the iris. Finally the lens may be placed in the anterior chamber (AC-IOL).

The miLoop© Recently, a device marketed as the *miLoop©* has been developed to assist in fracturing hard lens nuclei (Fig. 14.3). The functional element of this small handheld device is a flexible, retractable, nitinol loop (wire made of titanium and nickel) that is designed to engage the nucleus within the capsular bag, encircling it and, when retracted like a noose, sectioning the entire nucleus in two. The loop can be re-engaged multiple time, effectively sectioning the lens into smaller pieces.

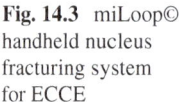
Fig. 14.3 miLoop©
handheld nucleus
fracturing system
for ECCE

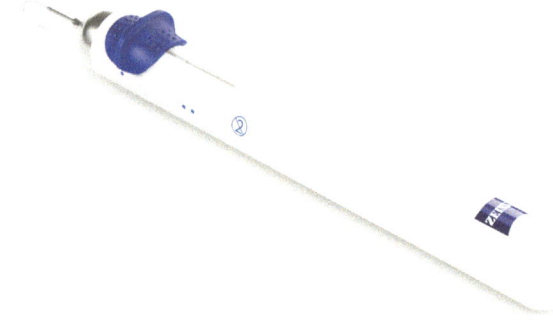

As a scrub you will find that there is virtually no unusual preparation required to hand off his device to the surgeon. The OR circulator will open the sealed package and transfer the sterile device to your table. Prior to using the miLoop, and after the capsule has been opened, the surgeon will hydrodissect the nucleus from the cortex using a saline syringe with a small-bore blunt cannula. Once the lens has been bisected using the miLoop(c) the phaco system is employed to complete the procedure.

Intracapsular Cataract Extraction

Where there are circumstances that suggest that the lens zonules are damaged or diseased beyond their capacity to maintain the stability of the lens during phaco-emulsification or ECCE, the surgeon may opt to perform an intracapsular cataract extraction (ICCE). This procedure includes the removal of the *entire cataractous lens* from the eye – capsule and all – resulting in a condition known as surgical apha-kia. There are two approaches to effectively removing and unstable lens from the eye.

ICCE: Anterior Approach

This procedure requires a large incision and often special tools such as a cryophake – a handheld device where the tip can freeze to the lens capsule and lifted from the eye. (Did you ever get your tongue stuck momentarily on a dry ice cube? Well, that's exactly the concept that your surgeon would use to remove the entire cataractous lens – nucleus, cortex, and capsule – with the cryophake.) (Fig. 14.4). The lens is now in a state of aphakia (without lens), and this leaves the surgeon staring through the microscope looking directly into the unadorned vitreous cavity. The vitreous, gel-like and mobile, now unimpeded by the intact lens, may be invited to

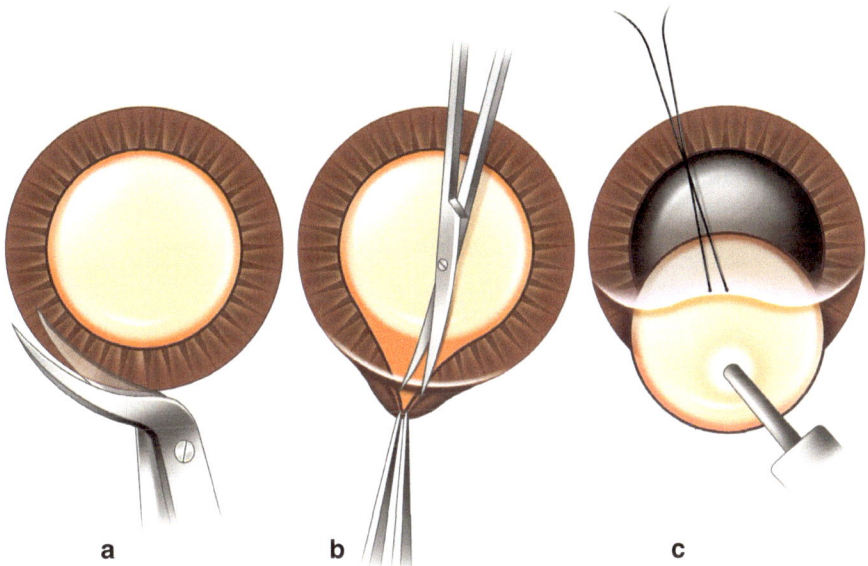

Fig. 14.4 Historic Intracapsular Cataract Extraction (ICCE) using cryo-extraction. (**a**) Micro-scissor corneal incision (**b**) Peripheral iridotomy (**c**) Extraction of entire, intact lens

move forward from the vitreous cavity toward the front of the eye (anterior chamber) and may encourage a number of hazards: Vitreous has an almost mystifying ability to find its way forward in the eye and is routinely found trapped in the corneal wounds days after surgery. In doing so vitreous may distort the pupil, decenter the lens implant, invite inflammation, and tears and detachments of the retina.

So, if vitreous is found in the AC, your surgeon may be required to perform an anterior vitrectomy (or occassionaly, depending on the surgeon's level of training and skills, a vitrectomy through the pars plana). In some cases where there is only a thin strand of vitreous trapped in the wound or otherwise causing concern your surgeon may use a micro-scissor – Vannas – to cut the strand and release the traction that might be applied to the retina by the perceived vitreous traction. If a vitrectomy is required you will be asked to break out the vitrectomy hand -piece. Thus is an additional standard piece of equipment inventoried in your ASC. The set up is similar to the phaco pak but the infusion and aspiration/cutter functions will be separated. The surgeon will placed the cutter through the main wound and the infusion hand-piece through the side port. Prior to inserting an IOL a small opening in the iris is often manufactured (iridotomy) (Fig.14.4) to insure that a lens implant (or occult vitreous) will not block the necessary migration of aqueous (manufactured in the area of the ciliary body) through the pupil and then into the anterior chamber, and finally out of the eye through the trabecular meshwork in the angle of the anterior chamber.

ICCE: Pars Plana Approach

The pars plana approach is like the pars plana approach for an ECCE, except here the retinal surgeon will vitrectomize the entire lens as well as clean the vitreous from the eye. The result is a condition where there is no secure capsular support and the implantation of an IOL takes on a completely set of unique options (Sutured or glued three piece PC-IOL or AC-IOL).

Chapter 15
Femto Laser-Assisted Cataract Surgery (FLACS)

For more than four decades, phaco – ultrasonic fragmentation of the lens – has been the standard for cataract surgery among developed countries. It was predictable, then, that eventually new technological innovations would give the cataract surgeon and their patients expanded options to cataract surgery. Recently a laser system – a *femto second laser* – was developed that performs multiple discrete procedures, both on the cornea and within the eye, that will assist the surgeon at cataract surgery before entering the eye.

But first, what is a "laser"? The word itself conjures up all sorts of fantasy weapons: just think of every Star Wars film you've ever seen and its imitators. The word laser is an acronym for *Light Amplification by Stimulated Emission of Radiation*. I can sense your eyes glazing over. But hold on, this gets easier.

Unlike light emanating from a simple light bulb – visible light – and able to provide light across a large area (think of your bedroom lamp), suffusing the entire room with light energy which, for the most part, has no immediate physical impact on anything in the room, a laser light is "coherent" and "directional" – collimated we call it – and the energy now bundled in this way can be used like a physical tool. Depending on the wavelength of the emitted light (determined by certain materials used as the excititory mechanism producing the defined light) a laser becomes a tool determined by the absorbtion spectrum of the targeted material (biologic in our case).

So, a laser can be fashioned, for example, for medical application into a *cold disrupting tool*, to, say, break anatomical structures apart – or a *heat producing, coagulating tool* – that would be applicable to sealing leaking blood vessels in the retina (typical of diabetic retinopathy). It all depends on the wavelength of the laser light and the absorption spectrum of the targeted anatomy.

A femto laser *tool produces* a coherent light at a wavelength that makes for a "cold" disrupting tool. When applied to certain eye tissues, it will produce exquisitely fine and perfectly positioned incisions without any collateral damage. The femto laser energy can be designed to disassemble or breakup lens material in predetermined patterns based on the surgeon's approach to the procedure. It does this leaving adjacent tissues uniquely undisturbed.

The entire package of procedures provides an assist to the phaco procedure sparing a human hand for significant critical elements of the surgery. The entire laser application is accomplished from outside of the eye needing only a clean room environment, using only eye drop anesthesia and the assistance of a scrub nurse. An anesthesiologist is not required.

Once the patient is settled onto the laser treatment table, a complete femto procedure – positioning the patient beneath properly and engaging the eye – takes a matter of minutes. The laser treatment itself takes only seconds. The femto laser can provide painless entry wounds through the cornea, perform a perfectly round opening into the cataractous lens (capsulotomy) with variations in diameter, partially disassemble (fracture) the lens nucleus using a menu of pre-programmed configurations, and treat astigmatism with arcuate incisions at the periphery of the cornea.

Once the femto procedure is completed, the patient is then brought to the standard OR where, under sterile conditions, the fractured nucleus is removed with the phaco handpiece, now requiring less phaco energy (heat) and manipulation – thus decreasing operative time and, practically speaking, potential risk.

Although there is a growing adoption of the femto techniques for routine cataract surgery, there are some reservations regarding its utility versus cost, since medical insurance does not cover the procedure. For the surgeon there is a comforting feeling sitting down at the operating microscope to complete a cataract procedure after a femto treatment where a perfect capsular opening has been fashioned; the lens is in an advantageous state of disassembly – requiring a shortened emulsification time; and the patient's astigmatism has been addressed. Is that enough reason to add the burden of expense to a patient's surgical care? We believe the decision to use the femto laser requires a candid discussion between surgeon and patient after providing all the facts germane to the technology.

In our practice we have found special utility for using femto technology where there are measured risks to prolonged intervention by standard phacoemulsification. These risks include disorders of the zonules, previous vitrectomy and retinal surgery, highly myopic eyes, advanced glaucoma, corneal endothelial disorders, and a history of significant blunt or intraocular trauma to the eye.

So, for those surgeons who consider that the femto laser is exquisitely more accurate than their own hand and equate shortening surgical time in the eye as mitigating risk, then the laser may justify its cost.

As a surgical scrub, you may or may not be trained on the femto laser system. Training differs depending on which manufacturer's device is purchased by your ASC. Since the laser will be placed in a separate room away from the OR, efficiency may dictate specific personnel to operate the laser, while the scrub nurse remains in the OR and prepares for the arrival of the patient from the femto suite.

The learning curve for assisting your surgeon during the femto procedure is relatively short, but requires attention to detail, something you have proven to be more than adept as you perform your surgical scrub skills. The femto manufacturer will spend as much time as necessary, over dry runs and actual surgery, to make you

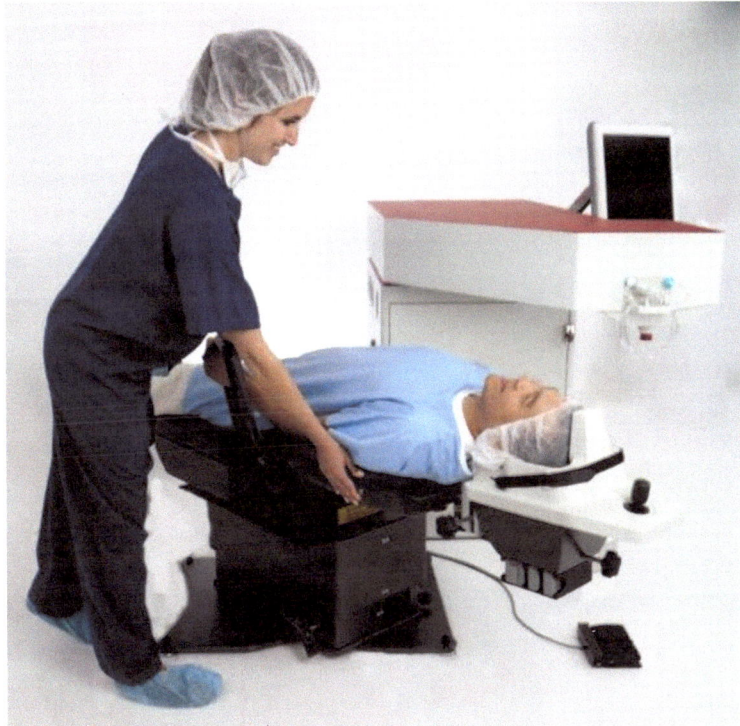

MK-00251 Rev A

Fig. 15.1 Patient being positioned on femto laser treatment table. (With permission of Johnson & Johnson)

comfortable going solo. The following is a short form of the femto laser procedure including both the surgeon's and scrub nurse's participation:

- A: The patient is positioned laying supine on the laser treatment table (Fig. 15.1). These tables may be mobile and used to morph into a chair-like system to move the patient from the laser suite once the procedure is completed or are stationery and integrated into the entire laser console, requiring a separate process to truck the patient to the standard OR.
- B: After a standard "time-out," the laser suction tubing and interface are assembled. This comes pre packaged and is placed into ports on the console.
- B: In some cases, a lid speculum may be used to keep the lids widely apart. After a drop of anesthetic is placed on the eye, the suction ring itself is positioned directly on the cornea with the assist of a computer monitor assisting in the "docking" process in real time.
- Figure 15.2 shows an overview of femto procedure.
- C: Careful centering of the laser on the cornea is important, and you will help guide the surgeon by describing what you view on the monitor, while the surgeon

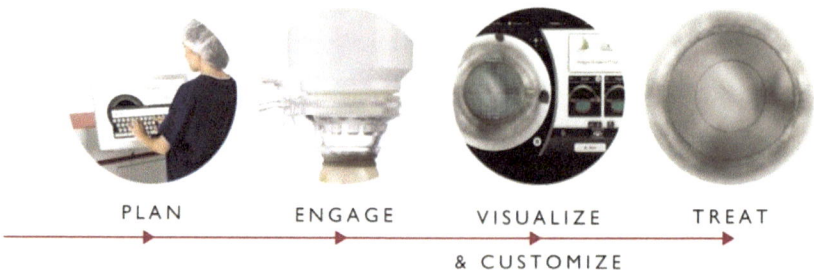

PLAN   ENGAGE   VISUALIZE   TREAT

& CUSTOMIZE

MK-00251 Rev A

Fig. 15.2 Overview of femto procedure. (With permission of Johnson & Johnson)

- Gentle dock for patient with minimal intraocular pressure (IOP) rise and minimal hemorrhaging
- No corneal distortion or induced folds
- Clear optical path for precise imaging and laser delivery

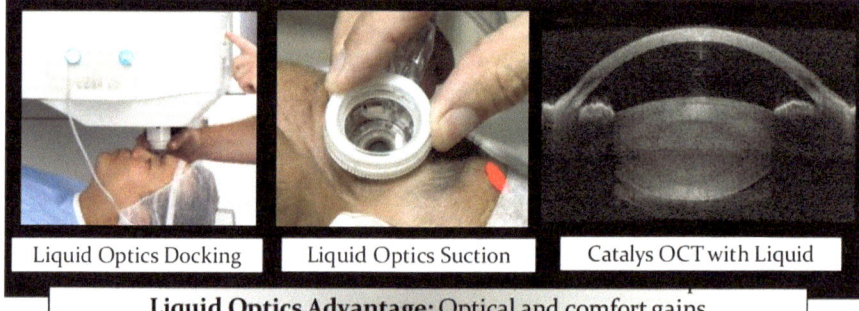

| Liquid Optics Docking | Liquid Optics Suction | Catalys OCT with Liquid |

Liquid Optics Advantage: Optical and comfort gains

MK-00251 Rev A

Fig. 15.3 Laser docking system and resulting imaging guidance on monitor. (With permission of Johnson & Johnson)

may be checking directly on the patient's eye. Once you and the surgeon have confirmed accurate placement of the suction ring, the surgeon will either use a foot pedal or joy-stick control to engage suction.

- Figure 15.3 shows a laser docking system and resulting imaging guidance on monitor.
- A. Once suction ring is engaged by the lens docking system, with the laser adequately centered as confirmed on the monitor (Fig. 15.4) – and depending on the design of the system – the surgeon or the surgical scrub will take the system

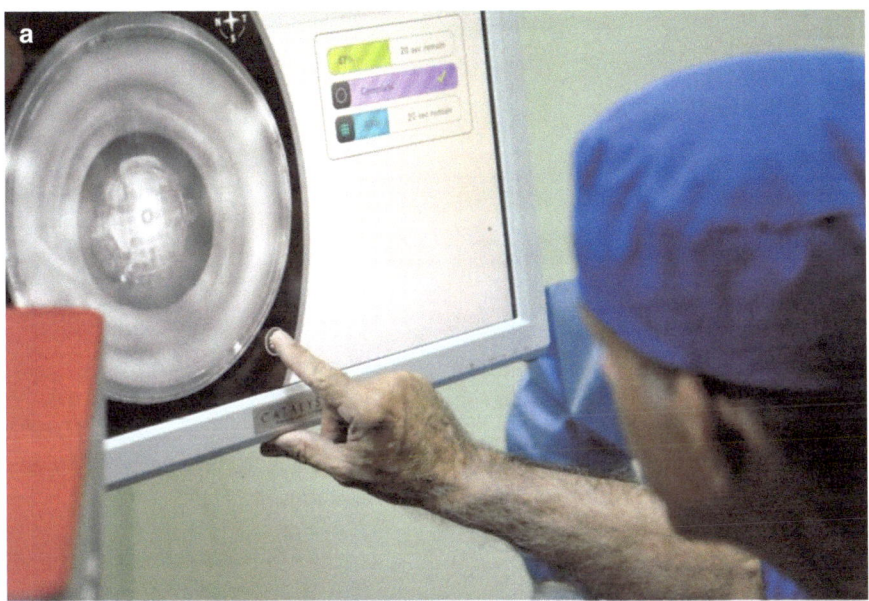

MK-00251 Rev A

Quick, template based planning performed prior to patient dock

MK-00251 Rev A

Fig. 15.4 (a, b) Femto monitor: data acquisition guidance prior to actual laser implementation. (With permission of Johnson & Johnson)

Fig. 15.5 Operating
microscope view of the
completed femto procedure
with arcuate corneal
incisions, laser
capsulotomy, and quadratic
disassembly of lens
nucleus. (With permission
of Johnson & Johnson)

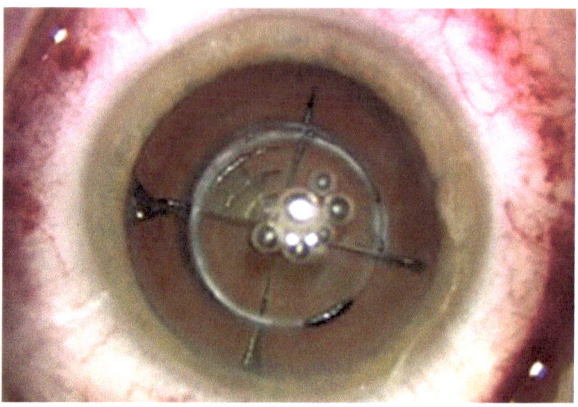

through a series of checks, which will include spacing the laser to interact within
the eye without causing damage to adjacent anatomic structures (for instance, the
laser application to the nucleus should not be so deep as to possibly penetrate the
back of the posterior capsule, leaving the nucleus to drop into the back of the eye).
- E. Once the procedure is completed, the suction device is removed and patient is
  either moved by chair or table to the OR (Fig. 15.5).

Chapter 16
Performing Phaco

Surgeons are often creatures of habit. Although a skilled phaco surgeon will bob and weave depending on the changing conditions they might face in the heat of battle – meaning they are adaptive and resourceful – when relatively relaxed and performing a rather routine case, you'll readily be able to predict what techniques they require at each step of the way. This works to your advantage since you will most assuredly have the correct instrument in your hand and ready to hand off before the surgeon requests them.

The following is a composite set of surgical directives and rituals that can be considered common to most surgeons:

Something to Consider Before Surgery If the patient has been scheduled for an astigmatic lens implant (called a toric lens), then your surgeon might consider marking the limbal region of the cornea across the 180 meridian in order to avoid "cyclotorsion" of the eye once they lay down. (The position of the eye may be altered simply by laying down.) The surgeon may perform this mark either free hand or using a toric marking system consisting of a ring marker with hash marks 360°, and a second instrument – the actual marking device – brushed with black ink that will leave a mark across the appropriate meridian at the limbus.

The Operation: Details

Before and during the surgery, you should make sure the cornea is kept moist (a dry cornea compromises the surgeon's visibility). Prior to surgery you might wish to ask the surgeon if they prefer that you drop sterile balanced salt solution (BSS) on the cornea when you feel it is necessary or wait for instructions from the surgeon.

© Springer Nature Switzerland AG 2020
R. S. Koplin et al., *The Scrub's Bible*,
https://doi.org/10.1007/978-3-030-44345-0_16

Positioning the Patient on the OR Table

Be sure that the patient is in a comfortable position; otherwise, they will begin to fuss during the procedure, attempting to find a position for their arm, legs, or back that is not stressed. Most importantly, unless instructed otherwise, position the patient's head so that the eye is *parallel with the floor*. Then have the patient look to the ceiling and consider how the lids (especially the upper) may be obstructing the surgeon's view of the entire cornea. Adjust the head using the knobs at the top of the table to raise or lower the head; this often repositions the eye in relation to the upper or lower lid. Occasionally you may have to instruct the patient to keep their chin slightly up or down to get this right. It is best to do this prior to performing the lid scrub.

Positioning the Operating Microscope

The operating microscope needs to meet several parameters for both the surgeon's comfort and function. Once it is determined whether the surgeon is operating from the side or from above — and which eye, left or right is to be operated — you should instruct the OR tech to position the microscope and phaco foot pedals under the table appropriately. Ask the surgeon on which side they want each of the foot pedals.

The OR tech should make sure that the microscope arm is strategically positioned so that when the X-Y coordinates (moving the oculars left, right and superiorly and inferiorly) are invoked there is enough running room to accommodate movement across the surgical field.

Once the surgeon is seated, they may ask to have the OR table raised or lowered to find a comfortable working distance from the eye or to position their legs beneath the table.

Entry into the Eye

When initiating the phaco procedure, your surgeon will usually make two entry wounds into the eye: both at the surgical limbus (where the clear cornea meets the white sclera), but there are variations on this theme. However, it is typical to make a main incision positioned for insertion of the phaco handpiece and at least one side port opening (also called a paracentesis or para) to assist with the second hand. Either of these openings can be made first:

- A thin blade approximating 15° as a cutting angle is often used to make one or more side port approaches. These will generally be made 3–4 clock-hours from the main incision.
- A trapezoidal or triangular blade (typically 2.2 mm, 2.4 mm, to 3.0 mm in width), called a keratome, is used to make the main surgical opening, usually fabricated

Fig. 16.1 Two entries
into eye

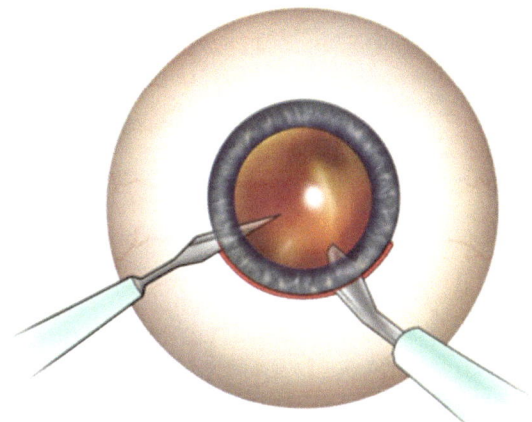

of metal or diamond material. Most surgeons operate from the temporal side (ear side) of the eye, while a smaller number operate from above, under the upper lid (Fig. 16.1). This also requires a seating adjustment for the surgeon, as well as turning the operating microscope to the desired position. Foot pedals – for both the operating microscope and phaco controls – must also be repositioned.

Stabilizing the eye to make an entry wound is a matter of preference. Some surgeons simply keep the eye immobilized with their index finger or a Q-tip, while others use various handheld instruments. Often these are finely toothed instrument forceps or in one case a ringlike fixation devices that circles the cornea which are relatively atraumatic and provides adequate stabilization while the surgeon's blade perforates the eye.

Some surgeons, although they use phaco, employ a scleral incision to enter the AC instead of a corneal approach. In this case the surgeon considers that the wound is more secure at the end of the procedure and therefore less likely to invite leakage and potential infection. The drawback is that more surgery is required. The conjunctiva must be incised, bleeding controlled with a micro-cautery, and often at the end of the procedure, the edges of the cut conjunctiva need to be re-apposed either with cautery or sutures. Although this technique is rarely used in western countries, it is commonly used where there are largely poor communities where ECCE (manual removal of the nucleus) is the less expensive than phaco and is therefore the treatment of choice.

Intraocular Anesthetics and Dilating Adjuncts

Often your surgeon will use 1 cc of 1% unpreserved lidocaine as an intraocular anesthetic. It may sting slightly for an instant when injected (usually through side port), and it is best to forewarn the patient. It is helpful in difficult cases where the surgeon either purposefully (patient with iris stuck to the lens – synechiae) or accidentally manipulates the iris. When filling the syringe from the drug vial held by a circulator (remember this is a sterile technique), you will use a 25 gauge needle, draw up the anesthetic, remove the needle, and replace it with a 25 gauge blunt cannula (not a sharp needle).

Be sure you have purged of any air from the syringe. (Position the syringe perpendicularly with the cannula side up, snap it with your finger to free the air from the sides of the plastic so that the bubbles rise to the top of the syringe, and then exit them by expressing the plunger less than a few tenths of a cc.)

Variations include the additional use of a dilating agent such as 1 ml of epinephrine hydrochloride 0.001% or Omidria (phenylephrine 1% and ketorolac 0.3% intraocular solution) injected into the AC after one or both incisions are made. Omidria is suggested in cases where you wish to prevent miosis (pupil becoming smaller). It is not as efficient as a solitary pupil dilator.

A combination of anesthetic and dilating agent is used commonly after femto laser procedures since the laser may irritate the iris which will often become acutely miotic. It is also indicated when patients are using oral Flomax (tamsulosin) for an enlarged prostate and the associated urinary frequency in order to counter the vexing ocular side effect of a floppy iris (IFIS) and miosis. The mixture is known as *Shugarcaine* (after the eye surgeon who popularized it) and is a mixture of 9 mL of BSS Plus with 4 mL of 1:1000 bisulfite-free epinephrine and 3 mL of 4% preservative-free lidocaine.

Viscoelastic

This material – often referred to an as ophthalmic viscosurgical device, or OVD – is typically a clear viscous-gel preparation used to inflate and stabilize the AC. Think of these as space occupiers. Although they are biodegradable, they are not intended to remain in the eye after surgery. They are slow to be cleared from the eye, and if a modest amount remains, they tend to cause painful elevation of eye pressure some hours after surgery. Often, in these cases, the surgeon is required to "burb" the eye of the viscoelastic the following day to lower the IOP.

If an instrument were to be placed into the AC at surgery without a viscoelastic material filling the anterior chamber, the chamber would likely collapse, with the cornea coming in rough contact with a surgical instrument. This would be potentially damaging to the corneal endothelium.

Viscoelastics are available in several branded variations and are chosen by your surgeon or ASC based on the perceived needs of the surgical procedure. Some viscoelastics are more cohesive, and a bolus (a decided "lump" of material) injected into the AC tends to move almost as a single entity. It is more easily removed from the eye when it's no longer needed. A dispersive type of viscoelastic may be more geographically driven around the AC, but conversely it may be more difficult to remove at the conclusion of the surgery. Some brands include a combination of both a dispersive and cohesive OVD.

The viscoelastic comes packaged in a transparent plastic syringe. You will be required to engage the cannula supplied in the package and to "prime" the product

Fig. 16.2 Viscoelastic. Delivery system (Photographer: Bob Masini)

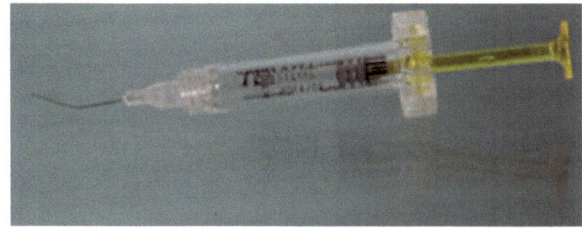

Fig. 16.3 Continuous curvilinear capsulorrhexis (CCC)

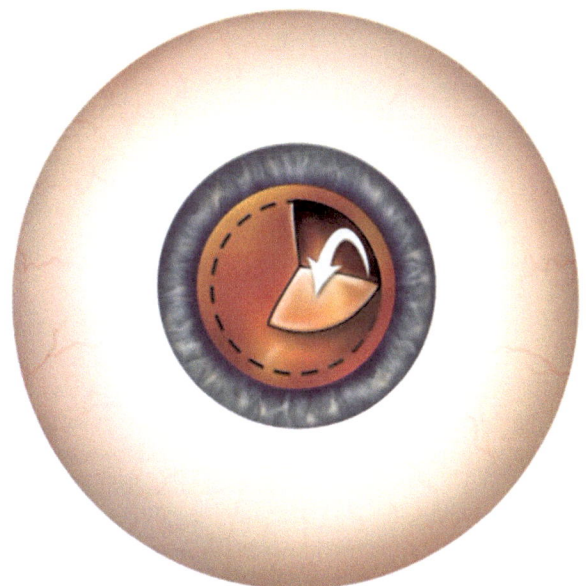

so air-bubbles do not enter the eye (usually expelling a small amount of the gel onto your gloved hand will do the trick). Lastly, before handing it off, reassure yourself that the cannula is securely fixed to the syringe.

The viscoelastic (Fig. 16.2) will be injected through one of the two openings (usually corneal) made by your surgeon. The remainder of the viscoelastic should be reserved for use in lubricating the lens implant when fitting it into the injector just prior to implantation and for the surgeon to reform the AC at the time of actual lens implantation.

Performing a Capsulotomy

The capsulotomy – a controlled, round tear in the front of the lens capsule – provides access to the lens nucleus (the central firm portion of the cataractous lens). Unless the capsulotomy was completed by a femto laser, the capsulotomy, known as a continuous curvilinear capsulorrhexis (CCC) (Figs. 16.3 and 16.4), will be

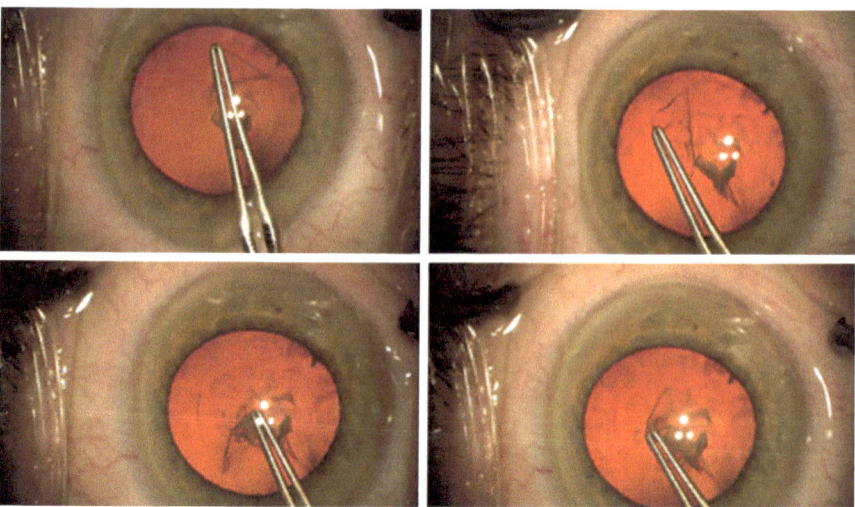

Fig. 16.4 Capsulorrhexis (panel of four images in sequence) (our stock image)

performed by your surgeon using several simple, handheld instruments. The average diameter of this circular opening may vary due to inherent restrictions related to the ability or inability to dilate the pupil fully and occasionally because of the fibrotic changes to the anterior capsule (where a microscissor may be required to complete the capsular opening). The average capsulotomy measures between 5 and 8 mm. The goal is not to leave any acute angles along the way that might tear out to the far periphery and make the nucleus vulnerable to a dislocation into the back of the eye.

A well-manufactured CCC leaves the nucleus and cortex bare to the phaco instruments with little chance of tearing out the anterior capsule.

To manufacture the CCC, a viscoelastic (OVD) will be used to fill the anterior chamber in front of the lens. The surgeon may enter the AC through one of the corneal openings with a bent needle (25 or 27 gauge) – called a cystotome – which will likely come packaged in the phaco kit purchased by your ASC. If necessary, you may manufacture the cystotome by using a needle holder to bend the tip of a 25 gauge needle and slightly angulate the shaft of the needle.

After making an initial tear on the anterior capsule, the surgeon will lift the edge of the capsule flap with special forceps (e.g., Utrata forceps) and manufacture the curvilinear tear for 360°. On rare occasions, you will find a surgeon who performs the entire capsulotomy by using the bent needle, pushing and pulling the capsular flap to complete a 360° opening.

Occasionally the capsulotomy may escape the surgeon's control and, as we say, "tear out." This means that the surgeon has lost control of the capsulotomy and a radial tear has begun to go further out toward the equator of the lens, threatening to tear beyond the zonules. This could cause the lens nucleus to dislocate into the vitreous or invite the vitreous into the AC if the surgeon should attempt to phaco the nucleus in this unstable situation.

In cases of a partial "tear out," the surgeon may ask for the return of the visco-elastic to flatten the lens capsule to control the tear and may then request a Vannas scissor or perhaps a long-armed microscissor to amputate (cut off) part of the run-away anterior capsule.

In some difficult cases where a CCC is not advisable or the capsule tears out, the surgeon may opt to perform a can-opener capsulotomy. This is manufactured by simply applying the bent needle to the periphery of the lens capsule in multiple short stabs toward the center. Moving circumferentially 360°, your surgeon will ultimately complete a central opening, albeit not one as smooth as a CCC and vul-nerable to tear-outs because of small acute angles oriented to the periphery.

If the patient has undergone a femto second laser capsulotomy, the patient will arrive in the operating room a few minutes after the procedure having undergone an astigmatic correction, possibly multiple entry wounds in the cornea. A perfectly round capsulotomy will be manufactured (known as a "cap.").

Occasionally the femto laser misses areas along the way (due to obscurations of the cornea, angulations of the eye, etc.), and the surgeon will be required to deli-cately complete the discontinuous portion(s) of the capsulotomy, careful not to tear the capsule out to the periphery and compromising the integrity of the entire "bag" (the term often used to describe the capsular element that surrounds the entire lens).

In all cases – femto, CCC, or "can-opener" – the surgeon will likely ask for an Utrata or toothed Kelman forceps to complete the removal of the "cap" from the AC under an appropriate OVD.

Hydrodissection and Hydrodelineation: Achieving Nuclear/ Cortical Separation

Using a 3 cc syringe filled with sterile saline, your surgeon will advance the blunt cannula beneath the anterior flap edge of the capsulorrhexis and gently deliver the saline under mild pressure in order to cleave the nucleus from the surrounding lens material and capsule. When successfully accomplished, this allows the nucleus to be mobilized and moved about with the phaco tip and accessory instruments.

Hydrodissection and hydrodelineation (Fig. 16.5) are potentially complicating if performed in cases where a *can-opener style capsulorrhexis* has been manufac-tured, since the advancing fluid wave may tear out the ragged edges of the anterior

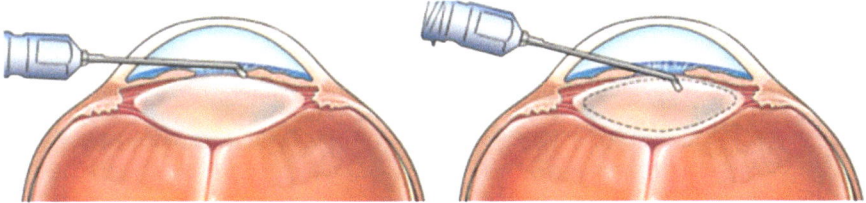

Fig. 16.5 Hydrodissection (left) and hydrodelineation (right)

capsule and continue the tear around and past the equator of the lens. If the surgeon is unaware of the tear there is the danger that further manipulation of the lens during phaco could drive the nucleus through the capsular tear and into the vitreous cavity.

Nuclear Disassembly The core concepts in lens removal in phaco surgery involve disassembling the approximately 10 mm round nucleus into smaller segments so that it can be removed through the much smaller 2.2 mm phaco needle port. This involves four basic themes:

Classic carousel cracking and emulsification (Fig. 16.6) Here the center of the lens is grooved with the console setting on "*sculpt*." (The console settings are often on the low side with modest vacuum and modest flow in sculpt mode.) The most popular technique requires that the nucleus be rotated, and at each quarter turn, the lens is grooved across the length of the nucleus resulting in a cross of sorts. Two instruments (often the phaco tip and a second instrument) are placed in the grooves and spread apart to separate or "crack" the nucleus, producing four relatively equal lens quadrants. Each quadrant is then emulsified with the console setting in the "*quadrant removal*" mode (Fig. 16.7). (Here the vacuum is increased, and the flow rate lowered for many surgeons.) Use the surgeon profile to engage the appropriate baseline settings. The surgeon will usually instruct you to adjust the settings – or move from aspiration to vacuum – higher or lower as needed.

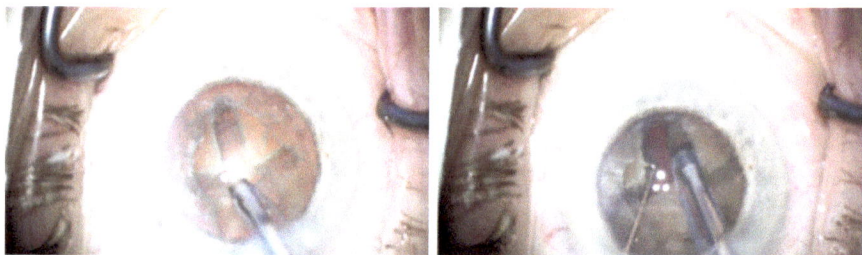

Fig. 16.6 Carousel cracking (two photos) (our stock image)

Fig. 16.7 Quadrant removal (our stock image)

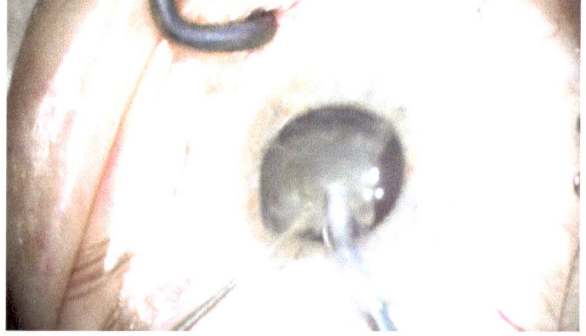

A second instrument is often essential in the various techniques for removing nucleus. This might be a spatula such as a *Drysdale spatula* or a hook such as a *Kuglen Hook*, which can act as a "pusher" or "puller" and is quite versatile.

Quadrant removal The settings will be altered when the surgeon moves to the next stage, which is generally, "*quadrant removal*," which often constitutes a higher vacuum with corresponding higher bottle height. The phaco tip is then used to draw up and emulsify the nuclear lens material segment by segment. You'll no doubt be witness to the rapidly evolving techniques and novel instrumentation in our field.

Phaco Chop: An Alternative to Carousel Cracking

With the console setting in "*chop*" mode or some variation (vacuum relatively high), your surgeon will impale the nucleus with the phaco-tip and use it to both stabilize and shift the lens slightly, to fit the chopper just behind the equator of the nucleus beneath the anterior leaf of the capsule. The chopper is then drawn toward the phaco tip to "chop" the nucleus. Alternatively, the phaco tip and the chopper are used to impale the nucleus a bit off the center. The chopper is twisted away from the phaco needle to crack a section of nucleus away. The lens is rotated and with each "chop" another discrete slice of nucleus is produced: each segment is then emulsified at a phaco setting appropriate to the perceived hardness of the lens.

There are dozens of choppers on the market. The choice is strictly a personal preference by your surgeon. These are variable in design, but all are designed to accomplish the same end.

Ultrasonic Power, Aspiration, and Vacuum These setting will be adjusted as the surgeon considers how dense the nuclear fragments might be and how mobile they are. Higher power or alterations in oscillatory and longitudinal needle movements are common.

Your surgeon may request resetting vacuum and/or aspiration where appropriate to both draw nuclear chips to the phaco tip and emulsify efficiently. Phaco needles may be straight or bent at the tip in several angled configuration. Interestingly the angulated 45° seems to be more efficient than a straight tipped phaco needle.

Epinucleus Removal Once the nucleus is fully emulsified and aspirated from the eye your surgeon will likely use the "*epinuclear*" mode to remove this shell of transitional lens material that resides *between* the nucleus and cortex. There is a pre-set for this function, so it is not likely you'll be required to change settings. The process employs very low power and vacuum settings, and modest aspiration. It is meant to friendly to the capsule and lessens the possibility of tearing it.

Irrigation and Aspiration: Cortical Cleanup Now that all the nuclear and epinuclear lens material has been removed, attention is turned to the soft, fluffy cortical material adjacent to the capsule.

Fig. 16.8 Cortical clean up (our stock image)

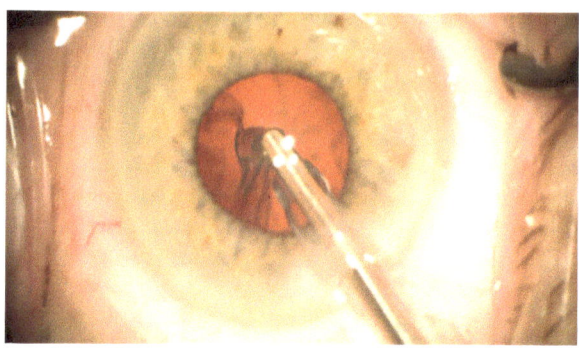

You will remove the infusion and aspiration lines from the phaco handpiece and place them on the IA handpiece. Press the appropriate menu button on the remote or have the circulator press the analogous button on the console for "*Cortex/IA.*" Once the infusion and aspiration line are attached and secure, remind your surgeon to step briefly on the foot pedal to clear any air bubbles prior to placing the instrument in the eye.

Depending on the ease of cortical removal, your surgeon may or may not ask for the aspiration rate to be raised or lowered. 25–35 cc per minute is an average setting in IA, but small increments can make for rather dramatic alterations in the aspiration mode and the stability of the AC. Surgeons must be careful regarding inadvertently aspirating the capsule. Your surgeon may ask for either a straight or curved I&A tip.

Figure 16.8 shows cortical clean up.

Capsule Polishing Often, at the conclusion of the IA portion of the procedure, your surgeon may request the "*polish*" setting on the I&A handpiece. This provides a gentle aspiration which facilitates removal of little plaques of adherent lens material to the posterior capsule and underside of the anterior capsular leaves. Alternatively, your surgeon may request a metal capsule polisher or the viscoelastic syringe (using the blunt cannula) to scrape clean the posterior capsule.

IOL Implantation Once the surgeon is comfortable that all lens fragments have been removed from the eye and the capsule is clear of debris, viscoelastic will be used to inflate the capsular bag and fill the anterior chamber. If an astigmatic IOL is to be inserted, it is here that the cornea will be marked at the appropriate axis using a toric marker (or remarked to confirm the axis indicated if there was a preliminary marking prior to initiating the procedure).

If your surgeon intends to use the ORA wavefront-guided lens confirmation system, it would occur at this point in the operation.

A detailed discussion of lens calculations, lens types, and implantation methods will be found in the following chapter.

Wound Closure Once the surgeon is satisfied that the lens is perfectly placed in the capsular bag, they will do one of the two things:

Consider that the wound is stable; they will request the IA handpiece, have the console setting on "*visco*" (*viscoelastic evacuation*), and then remove viscoelastic and very small particles of lens from the AC.

Your surgeon will then commonly request saline in a 3 cc syringe with a blunt cannula and then hydrate the edges of the main corneal wound and side port. By forcing fluid into the stroma at the wound edges, the swollen cornea will force the wound closed (Fig. 16.9). Drying the wounds with a mini-sponge will further assure that wound is tight.

The surgeon will then test the eye pressure by gently tapping the eye (experience gives inference to what is normal and what is not), and if the surgeon feels that eye

Fig. 16.9 Hydrating wound (our stock image)

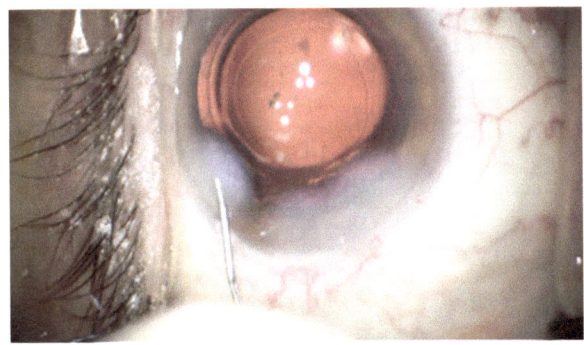

Fig. 16.10 Loaded needle holder: (Photographer: Bob Masini)

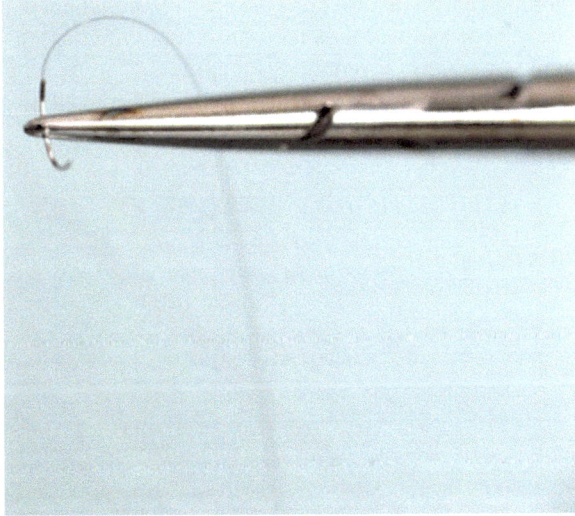

is over-infated they will "burp" the side port to release a small amount of fluid and if too soft, re-inflate the eye.

Alternatively, consider that the wound may not be competent; your surgeon will place a single suture through the center of the main wound. If this is the case, you will prepare a single-armed 10-0 nylon suture on a needle holder (Fig. 16.10). Take care unwinding the nylon suture material from the package since it is easy to catch and break the suture or tear the needle away from the nylon.

A microneedle holder is used to grasp the needle just behind mid-shaft. Hand it to the surgeon so that they may keep the jaws firmly closed around the needle (especially if it is a non-locking instrument). As you hand this to your surgeon, it is good form to announce that the needle holder is either *locking* or *non-locking*, meaning when you close the arms of the forceps a catch maintained the arms closed without pressure (locking) or there was no such mechanism (non-locking) and the surgeon must maintain pressure on the arms of the forceps or risk dropping the needle. The surgeon will then request a fine-toothed forceps to hold the lips of the wound in order to pass the needle. Finally, your surgeon will request a Vannas scissor to trim the suture ends and then use one of the two tying forceps to bury the knot.

A Word About Sutures Suture diameter or thickness is designated by a set of numbers, along with the material. The higher the number, the thinner the suture material. So, a suture designated *10-0 nylon* is thinner – lesser diameter – than *9-0*. Cataract surgeons commonly work with 10-0 nylon; however under certain conditions, the surgeon may use Prolene or Vicryl sutures for other chores.

If a suture is to be placed (but not tied), it may be best to do this when the eye is still filled with viscoelastic. Doing this is more efficient since once the OVD is removed, the AC may be unstable and readily collapse. Once the suture is passed through cornea and sclera – *untied* – the surgeon will evacuate the AC with the I&A handpiece and will then request a set of tying forceps to secure the suture. Usually only one suture is required (Fig. 16.11). The surgeon will use the tying forceps to rotate the knot into the wound (left unburied the knot will irritate the patient).

Fig. 16.11 Wound 10-0 nylon suture buried (rotated) into corneal wound (our stock image)

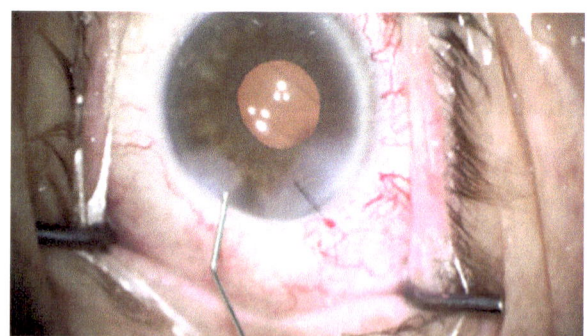

Fig. 16.12 Super Scrub is expert with a needle and thread

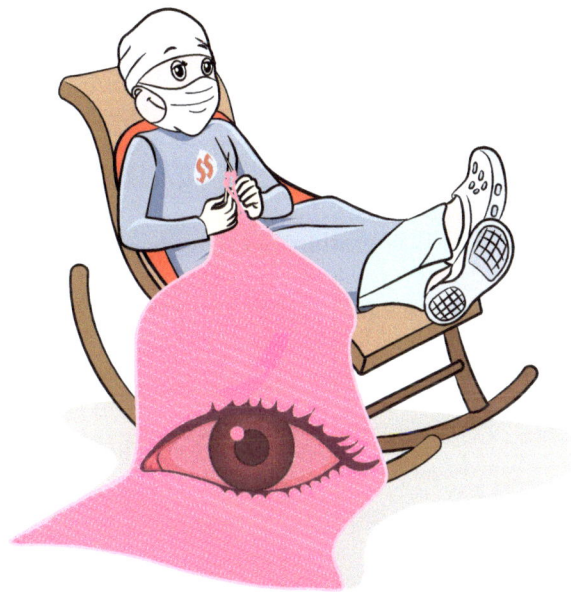

Occasionally your surgeon will accidentally break the suture as they are tying or attempting to bury it, and they will be required to repeat the process. Unfortunately, if the patient has not been blocked, they will feel a slight "pinch" as the needle is passed (Fig. 16.12).

Finally, the surgeon will once again confirm that the eye is not over or under inflated.

Concluding the Procedure

At the conclusion of the phacoemulsification procedure, the eye is generally washed with antibiotic and corticosteroid solutions. Some surgeons prefer an antibiotic ointment.

Shield, Patch, or Plastic Wraparound Sunglass The patient will usually leave the operating room with some sort of protective gear; this is the surgeon's choice. Most surgeons will use a clear shield taped to the face with hypoallergenic tape. The patient will be instructed to wear the shield overnight, until they see their surgeon the next day. In some cases, a wraparound sunglass is supplied. In some cases the surgeon will instruct the patient to carefully place prescribed eye drops in the operated eye on a schedule supplied by the surgeon. In other cases the surgeon will take a conservative approach and ask the patient not to remove the patch or shield (if there is one) and wait until they are seen by the surgeon for their first post operative evaluation.

Some surgeons apply a full patch with tape to cover the eye. This is more common when the patient is given a peribulbar block because the normal blink reflex is interrupted for some hours and the eye will dry out without the lid firmly closed over the eye.

At this point the patient is assisted from the surgical suite to the recovery area, commonly in a wheel chair. The patient will be placed in a comfortable chair, and their vital signs will be checked periodically until stable, usually about half an hour. The patient will be provided light refreshments (e.g., juice and a muffin) and allowed to leave the ASC with assistance.

You have just scrubbed on an uncomplicated phacoemulsification procedure. But life is not always a bed of roses.

Chapter 17
Lens Implants and Implantation: Determining Lens Power and Design

Understanding Farsighted and Nearsighted Eyes and How Your Surgeon Makes an Implant Choice

When considering a cataract extraction, certain IOL measurements are required to assure a satisfactory surgical outcome. Virtually all cataract procedures require a lens implant. After all, your surgeon is going to remove the patient's biologic lens, and a replacement lens of an appropriate power – calculated to the patient's needs – is paramount. This depends not only upon the surgeon's selection but also your confirmation that an IOL of the correct power is brought into the operating room.

Before discussing IOL power further, we need to first understand how a lens functions to assist in the process of "vision." The eye acts much like a camera. Not so much like a modern digital or phone camera but like an old-fashioned camera (called a single lens reflex camera – SLR) where there is a real lens and film (akin to the retina). The lens focuses or bends light rays from an image onto a point on the film. Each lens has a "power" which refers to its ability to bend light. Power is expressed in "diopters." A lens with a higher power can bend light more strongly (acutely) than a lens with a lower power.

A patient who is nearsighted usually has a long eye and requires a lens of low power to correct it to accurate distance vision without a residual prescription, while a farsighted eye is often relatively short and requires a high-powered lens to place an image on the retina (film).

Figure 17.1 is a schematic of an emmetropic, a myopic, and a hyperopic eye.

So, the need for glasses after a cataract operation (Fig. 17.2) will be determined first by what the patient desires as an outcome. Do they want to see distance without the aid of glasses and just wear reading spectacle or just the opposite? Once the decision is made, biometric measurements are performed which give options that are usually very accurate, but not perfect. And then there is biology. Every patient

© Springer Nature Switzerland AG 2020
R. S. Koplin et al., *The Scrub's Bible*,
https://doi.org/10.1007/978-3-030-44345-0_17

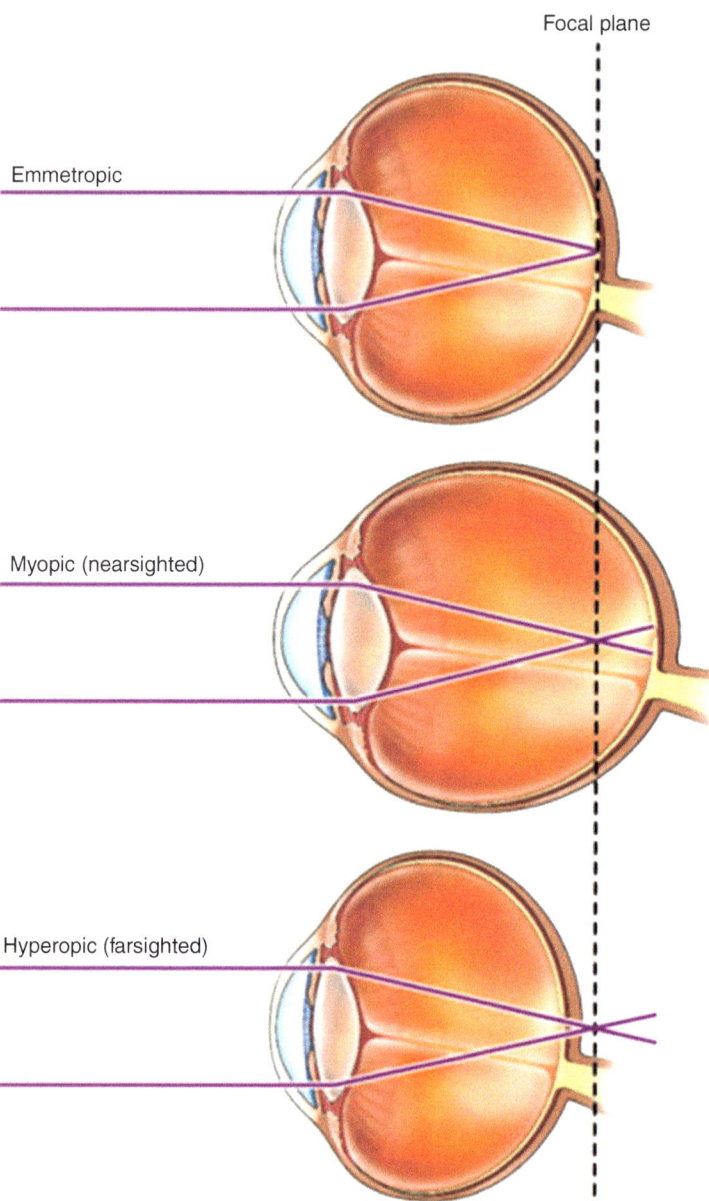

Focal plane

Emmetropic

Myopic (nearsighted)

Hyperopic (farsighted)

Fig. 17.1 Schematic of emmetropic, myopic, hyperopic eye

heals differently, and the final position of the lens implant, once all healing is accounted for, might find the lens a fraction of an inch further toward the front or the back of the eye resulting in a refractive error of some degree. That's the luck of the draw. Ordinarily the error is small.

Fig. 17.2 Super Scrub
wearing glasses

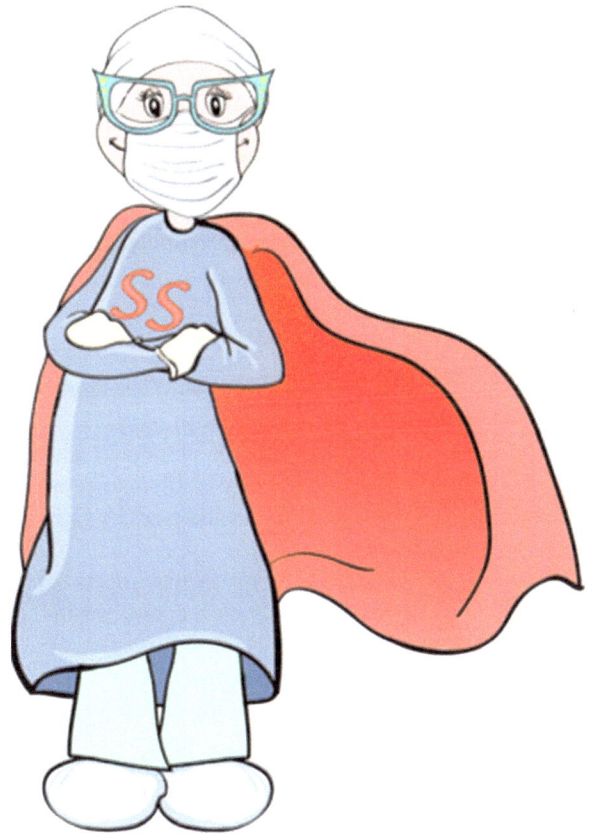

The correct IOL power selection depends on accurate measurements of two biometric data elements:

1. The length of the eye, also called axial length
2. The power of the cornea curvature

Calculating and choosing the appropriate IOL for a patient requires technology and consideration to the patients pre-surgical optical status, their vocation — if still working — as well as hobbies, sports, disabilities, etc. An IOL that does not meet the patient's needs may require surgery to exchange the lens.

Once at the ASC, choosing the correct lens implant and delivering it to the operating suite is the responsibility of your surgeon, but there is a sense of team work here. Prior to initiating surgery, the OR circulator will call for a "time out." At this point the patient and the eye to be operated upon will be confirmed as well as the power and style of the lens to be implanted, along with its expiration date. Additionally, the surgeon's list of lenses for the day should be available in the OR suite usually taped to the wall near the head of the operating table. Verbal confirmation should be made, and any vagaries clarified before beginning surgery.

Biometry: Assuring that the Correct Power Lens Implant Is Chosen

The required data needed to make the calculations are only two:

1. Length of the eye (axial length) measured from the front surface of the cornea to the surface of the retina.
2. The curvature of the front surface of the cornea measured, using a nomenclature called diopters. The corneal measurement, in this case, is a power-based calculation where the steeper the cornea, the greater the light bending capacity of the cornea.

Computations were originally based on regression analysis. This is basically using a crude algorithm (formula) or program and tweaking it by using the accuracy (or inaccuracy) of the outcomes of many past cases – experiential – as a guide to refining the algorithm. It's akin to a rifleman attempting to hit the bulls eye. After many misses to the left the marksman would logically adjust the rifle to the right. Its sort of empirical at first, but if you could actually make millimeter calculations over a large number of attempts the marksman's accuracy would increase. Similarly with IOL calculations; the more experience, as measured by a review of a large number of cases where the expected calculated (predicted) post operative outcome is compared to the actual outcome, can result in a correction factor that allows us to inch up to increasingly better patient satisfaction. In most cases a number of algorithms can be developed, each directed to the unique condition of a specific eye. As an example one formulation may work best for long eyes (myopes) and others may be found best for short eyes (hyperopes).

The ORA system: Prior to inserting a lens implant, your surgeon may use a technology meant to give added confidence to the choice of lens power or lens orientation. The device is used intraoperatively as a real-time measurement tool. The front end (the optical measuring device) is attached to the operating microscope and uses a Bluetooth connection to a floor-mounted monitor that guides the surgeon through the process of confirming data acquisition.

The ORA System™ (Optiwave Refractive Analysis) is meant to assist your surgeon by using an advanced optical technology that may provide a more secure estimation of IOL power and implant positioning. It is meant to be an adjunct to the surgeon's preoperative biometric calculations. The technology uses something called a wavefront aberrometer in which the optical wavefront from the device passes through a series of manipulations which analyze the many possible imperfections in the way light passes through the eye to the retina. So, the ORA may be able to confirm if the eye is in focus at the time of surgery, and if it is not, the surgeon is able to use the ORA System™ to refine the focus of the eye. In doing so the ORA may suggest adjusting the lens power or orientation.

So, depending on the surgeon's level of confidence in the predictive nature of their biometrics or, alternatively, the ORA data output, they may opt to use the lens implant they arrived with or ask for an ORA suggested lens power or orientation.

Using the ORA does cause inefficiencies in the OR, but some surgeons believe the effort is well worth it, while others are not so sure.

Lens Implant Design and Placement

The most common *intraocular lens (IOL) implant* used in uncomplicated phaco-emulsification surgery is a *posterior chamber lens (PCIOL)*. These lenses are designed to be placed within the capsular bag. If the capsular bag is not intact or there is zonular instability (tears may be in the anterior capsular or posterior capsule), the style of lens implant and whether it is a "firm" plastic or three-piece lens or soft foldable soft plastic will be considered as options.

Plastic/acrylic PCIOLs come in two basic designs: *three-piece* and *one-piece*.

1. *The three-piece implant* is of an older technology (not necessarily inferior, just different). The lens optic portion is manufactured of a foldable or solid plastic polymer or rarely a silicone material. Typically, there are two polymethyl methacrylate (PMMA plastic) *haptics 180 degrees from one another*, which are like wiry little elbows that jut out from the optical portion of the lens. The haptics are the stabilizing devices that keep tension against the inside of the lens capsule and maintain the lens centration.

   Three-piece implants are used mainly for placement in the ciliary sulcus (where the capsular bag may be unstable – torn zonules, perhaps – or not totally intact) (Fig. 17.3). Alternatively, three-piece implants are sutured to the iris or fixed in the sclera using the sutures tied to the haptics. Using a biologic glue and sclera pocket has become a popular alternative to suturing to the sclera.

2. *The one-piece implant* design is a soft (easily foldable) acrylic material with haptics that are continuous with the design and material of the optical portion of the lens (Fig. 17.9). It is an advanced technology since the material allows for a centered lens within the capsular bag, but it does so without the springy character of the PMMA haptics noted with the three-piece lens (Fig. 17.4).

   The one-piece design is not generally recommended outside the capsular bag, but this is the surgeon's choice.

Fig. 17.3 A three-piece IOL placed in the ciliary sulcus

Ciliary sulcus fixation

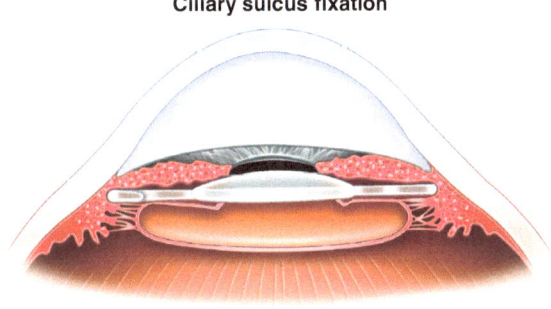

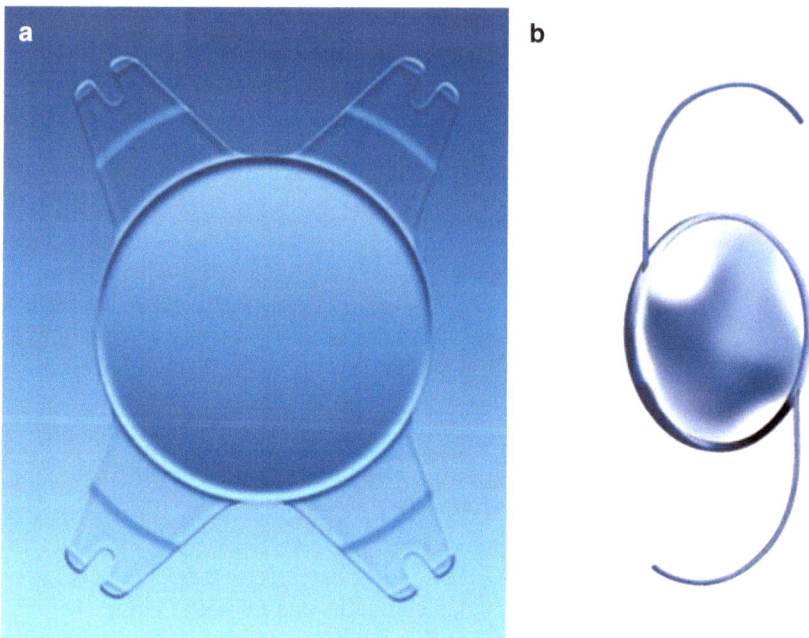

Fig. 17.4 (**a**) One-piece lens with four stabilizing haptics (**b**) three-piece lens with spring-like haptics. (Courtesy of Bausch and Lomb)

Fig. 17.5 Lens implant is completely within the intact capsular bag after uncomplicated phaco

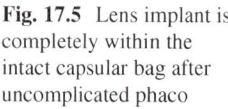

In-the-bag fixation

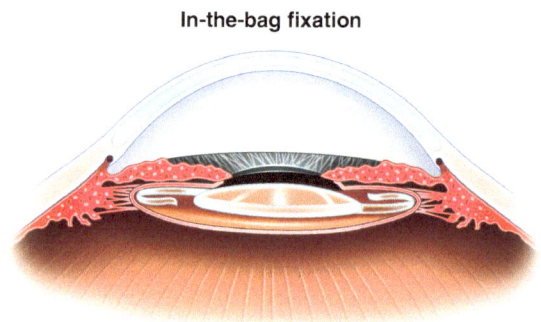

The soft acrylic lenses have garnered the moniker "the gummy-bear" implants because of their soft, pliable texture and slow unfolding optic and haptics after insertion into the capsular bag. The insertion process for both three piece and single piece are not dissimilar; however the three-piece haptics tend to open more abruptly. The single-piece soft foldable lens opens gradually. The unfolding process occasionally requires some gently manipulation to assure that the haptics don't stick to the optic portion of the lens (Fig. 17.9). A PMMA haptic associated with the three-piece lens may open quickly and in a compromised situation (as in a shallowing anterior chamber) may result in a tearing the anterior capsule or cause injury to the corneal endothelium.

Figure 17.5 shows a lens implant completely within the intact capsular bag after uncomplicated phaco.

Another lens design is called an *anterior chamber lens* (*ACIOL*). When a phaco-emulsification procedure goes without complication, there is little reason to implant anything but a PCIOL. An ACIOL is an option when there is concern for the integrity of the capsule or zonules—and therefore the ultimate stability of a lens implant if it were to be placed in the capsular bag or ciliary sulcus.

So, in those cases where the capsular bag is compromised, the surgeon may opt to place a lens in the anterior chamber, i.e., in front of the iris. All AC-IOL's are one piece and made of a firm PMMA material. The insertion may be assisted using a device called a *Sheets Glide*, a thin piece of plastic measuring about 15 mm by 6 mm that allows the surgeon to slide the lens down the glide securely into the anterior chamber.

Lens Implantation with Loss of Capsule Support:

Since there are no anatomical fixation opportunities existing in the posterior chamber where a surgery has lost the advantage of "in the bag" support, your surgeon will contemplate one of the following procedures to provide the patient with a satisfactory pseudophakic (lens implant) outcome:

A. *Anterior chamber lens implant*: placed in the angle of the anterior chamber in front of the iris (Fig. 17.6).
B. *Iris sutured three-piece implant*: the lens implant is stabilized by two sutures beneath the mid-iris and circled around the lens haptics. A downside is often the inability to fully dilate the pupil.
C. *Sutured three-piece posterior chamber lens implant*: sutures placed through the sclera at the pars plana to attach to three-piece implants once it is inserted in the appropriate position within the eye. The sutures are often buried beneath the sclera.

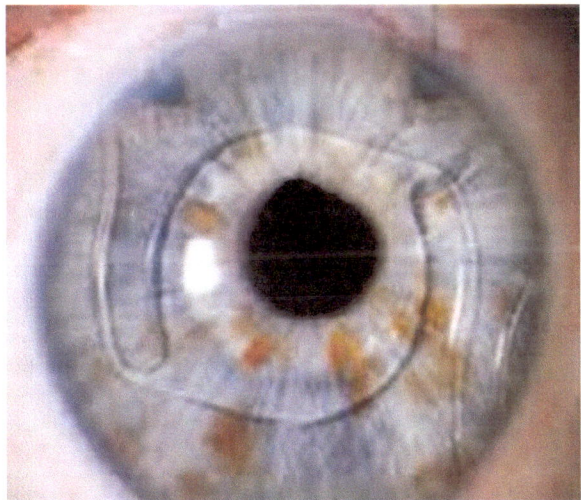

Fig. 17.6 Anterior chamber lens, placed in front of iris and quite visible to the examiner

D. *Glued posterior three-piece chamber lens implant*: here scleral pockets are manufactured 180 degrees from one another, and the lens – once inserted – is manip-
ulated so that the flexible haptics are each buried within the scleral pockets and
biocompatible glue applied over the lens haptics for further stability.

Premium Lens Implants

Multifocal, Extended Range and Toric Lens Implants

The "standard" lens implant, which has a "fixed focus" is the most common implant
used in the cataract surgery. It is safe and effective, but once implanted, the patient
would be capable of seeing well at only one distance – usually a choice made by the
surgeon in consultation with their patient; near or distance are the most common
choices, but anything in between is fair game. However, there are newer intraocular
lens technologies known as a family of premium *lens implants* that offer patients a
broader range of options. These lenses more aggressively speak to the patient's
multifocal or astigmatic needs. They are marketed as "multifocal" or "extended
range" products in combination or independently with astigmatic technology. So,
these implants have moved us one step closer to a form of "natural" vision; the goal
is to eventually free cataract patients from spectacle (glass) correction entirely.

Astigmatic correcting lens implants – available in combination with multifocal
or extended range implants – is a rather mature technology that is capable of neu-
tralizing most of a patient's astigmatism. Astigmatism is a condition where the corneal shape is less than appropriate for an idealized visual outcome.

Astigmatism occurs when the corneal curvature is steeper in one axis than
another (looks like a football). The condition is not a disease but can often cause
patient distress since their glasses must fit solidly on their face. Patients wearing
astigmatic spectacle corrections are often readjusting their glasses with the slightest
change in attitude of the lens placement. Implanting what is called a toric lens
(astigmatic) will relieve patients of most, if not all, of their astigmatic needs.

When using an astigmatic implant, your surgeon may be required to mark the
corneal axis prior to the patient lying down on the OR table. Marking the patients
presumed axis of astigmatism when sitting up avoids any change in the torqueing of
the eye when lying flat on the OR table. You will also require access to special axis
marking instruments prior to lens insertion. You should confirm that these instruments are available when you set up your surgical table.

The good news for you is that more than 90% of these lenses are set up in their
delivery systems no differently than a standard lens, so no concerns in this
department.

Much of the success of refractive implants is due to the work your surgeon
invests in the patient's careful clinical work-up and implant calculations prior to
surgery – and especially the choice of patient. Additionally, cataract removal must
be uncomplicated to safely implant a refractive lens. These lenses require precise

centering and should rarely be placed in the face of a torn capsule, or significant zonular disruption.

Admonition: We suggest that you take added care *not* to scratch these lenses on setup. Handle the central portion of the optic gently and as little as possible. A blemish in the center of a premium lens may – rightly or wrongly – be associated with a patient's postoperative complaints.

Insertion of a Posterior Chamber Lens

Posterior chamber lenses (PC-IOL) insertion: A foldable one-piece PCIOL must be loaded into a uniquely designed delivery system (a cartridge and *injector*) The cartridge with the lens placed inside is fitted to the injector (Fig. 17.7). Each manufacturer's delivery system is somewhat different. This is not meant to deliberately torture you, it simply has to do with the patent claims each company uses to forge their own unique IOL delivery system into the market.

The basic lens insertion system requires that you fill the cartridge included with the IOL product with the viscoelastic, and place the implant within the cartridge according to the manufacturers directions, assuring yourself that the haptics are folded appropriately. The cartridge is then placed onto the inserter. Most inserters use a screw system to deleliver the IOL into the eye. Manufacturers also supply preloaded implants.

Once the lens is fully inserted, hold he lens inserter up to the light and screw the mechanism a few turns to confirm that the lens is folded properly and moving forward without obstruction.

You will most likely have specially designed forceps on your tray to facilitate placing the lens into the IOL injector. You will be required to become familiar with the various inserters for each manufacturer. This is easier than it sounds, and you will meet this challenge in no time.

Figure 17.8 Super Scrub enjoys sliding into the eye on the lens inserter — the lens is smaller than a finger tip.

To ensure proper lens placement, hold the injector up to the light and scrutinize the lens, assuring yourself that it is sitting in the injector properly (i.e., make sure the haptics are folded just right and the lens is oriented properly). If you are in doubt, you can remove the lens and perform this ritual all over again. And, if necessary, ask the circulator for another vial of viscoelastic.

Fig. 17.7 Posterior chamber lens inserter. Metallic, reuseable. (Photographer: Bob Masini)

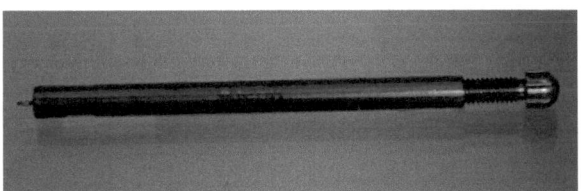

Fig. 17.8 Super Scrub enjoys sliding into the eye on the lens inserter — the lens is smaller than a finger tip

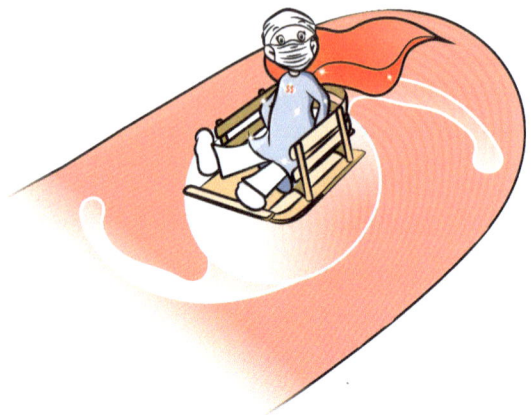

Where a three-piece foldable lens is to be used, it is likely that the surgeon has experienced a complication related to the capsule or zonules. Or, they may simply be suspicious that the stability of the capsule is questionable. In either case if the surgeon feels comfortable that there a suffcent support for the implantation of a posterior chamber lens it will likely be inserted in the ciliary sulcus taking advantage of the small incision. Alternatively, a surgeon may opt to open the wound to 6–7 mm and insert the lens unfolded and then close the wound with one or two 10-0 nylon sutures.

Where a *solid* acrylic lens is to be used (where the condition of the capsule may be suspect) the surgeon will open the corneal wound to approximately 7 mm, using a #15 blade, keratome, or curved corneal scissor, and insert the solid IOL using a Kelman-McPherson forceps, maneuvering the lens directly beneath the iris and into the ciliary sulcus.

Insertion of an Anterior Chamber Lens

Anterior chamber lenses (AC-IOL) insertion: An AC-IOL is often inserted where the capsule is so disrupted that it cannot lend any support to a posterior chamber positioned implant. Once the phaco and I&A are completed and any other procedures – such as a vitrectomy and a peripheral opening in the iris (peripheral iridotomy: a PI) to prevent a blocking fluid movement in and out of the eye are completed) a simple piece of thin plastic – known as a *Sheets Glide* – measuring 12 × 6 mm will be placed across the anterior chamber into the angle and it will be used by the surgeon as a glide to place the AC-IOL.

The wound will be enlarged to approximately 7 mm and the glide placed in the angle across the pupil and the AC-IOL placed in the angle while the glide is removed. Using forceps or Kuglen Hook, the trailing haptic is dropped into the angle just

Fig. 17.9 Manipulation of one piece foldable IOL into capsular bag using a Kuglen hook (our stock image)

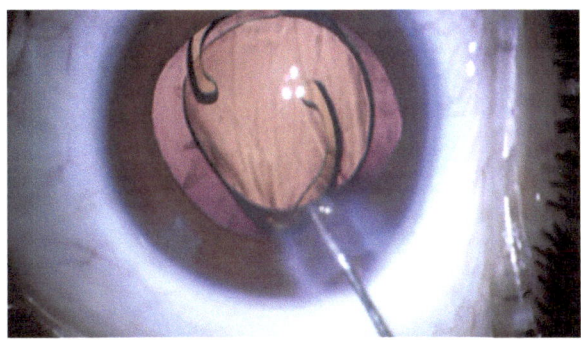

beneath the wound. Generally, several 10-0 nylon sutures are required to close the enlarged wound.

Timing: During the final minute or so of the I&A might be an appropriate time to ask your surgeon if you may go forward with loading the lens implant into its inserter. The reason you will ask this question, instead of simply going forward unannounced, is to provide the surgeon a moment of contemplation regarding any change in plans relative to the lens type. This happens occasionally if the surgeon should note a change in the integrity of the capsule at the conclusion of the cortical cleanup. This observation might lead your surgeon to consider altering the location of the intended implant, and this may entail a change in the lens design from, say, a single-piece soft acrylic lens to a three-piece lens with PMMA haptics or even solid plastic lens.

The fit diameters of the far end of the plastic lens inserter come in various sizes. Injectors are chosen depending on the type of lens to be inserted and will be accomodated through corneal wounds measuring 2.3–2.7 mm. If your surgeon believes that they may struggle with the fit of the lens injector, they may ask for a blade (15 degree or keratome) to slightly enlarge the wound.

Even a somewhat enlarged wound – if well designed – can be watertight after the conclusion of the procedure.

Occasionally, a lens implant haptic, or in some cases the lens optic, gets hung up in the wound, and your surgeon will request a tool – usually a *Kuglen or Sinskey hook* to manipulate the lens implant into final position (Fig. 17.9).

Chapter 18
Glaucoma Treatment as an Adjunct to Cataract Surgery

The Advent of MIGS

Glaucoma? Cataracts? How did we segue to glaucoma surgery from cataract surgery? Well, a funny thing happened on the way to refining microsurgery of the eye where a patient has both a cataract and a need for surgery and has experienced ongoing medical treatment for glaucoma.

Glaucoma is a disease most often associated with elevated eye pressure and you should think of it as a spectrum of disorders of the eye that have one thing in common: damage to the optic nerve. In most cases this nerve insult is related to a measurably elevated intraocular pressure (IOP), although exceptions exist (meaning patients can accumulate nerve damage with what are historically normal eye pressures).

Elevated IOP is secondary to fluid pressure. Aqueous fluid is manufactured by ciliary body, a muscular elevation that circles the internal portion of the eye just a few millimeters behind the lens. The newly secreted aqueous migrates forward around the lens periphery, through the pupil, and leaves the eye through a meshwork of tissue known as the filtering angle at the far edges of the insertion of the iris (360 degrees around the eye) and into the blood vessels adjacent to this area of anatomy (Fig. 18.1).

Although there are rather highly invasive surgical procedures to bring IOP down to levels that are meant to prevent progressive optic nerve damage, for the most part IOP is controlled with topical medications (eye drops) and occasionally laser treatments to the filtering angle to increase aqueous facility of outflow.

With the advent of innovative surgical technologies to treat glaucoma with minimal risks, there has been a tremendous growth of a procedure known as Microinvasive Glaucoma Surgery (MIGS). The surgery employs small "stents" – a few millimeters in length – that may be inserted into the filtering angle (usually the trabecular meshwork) at the time of cataract surgery (Fig. 18.2). There are several different stent

© Springer Nature Switzerland AG 2020   103
R. S. Koplin et al., *The Scrub's Bible*,
https://doi.org/10.1007/978-3-030-44345-0_18

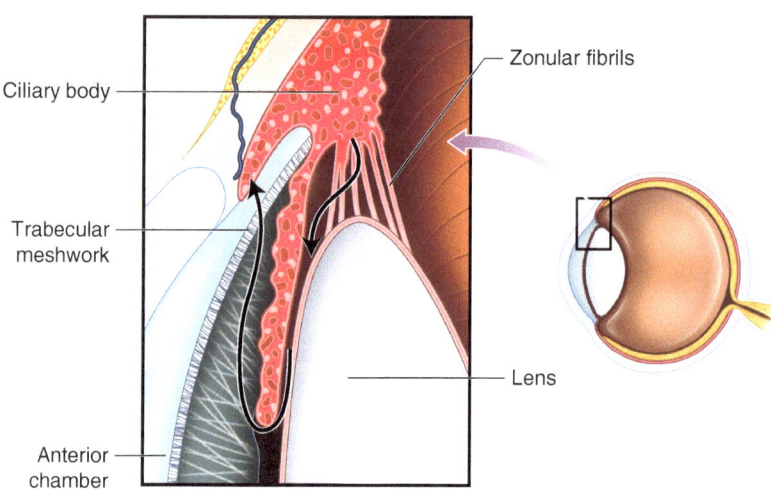

Fig. 18.1   Flow of Aqueous humor from ciliary body through trabecular meshwork

Fig. 18.2 (**a**) Micro stent positioned (**b**) handheld MIGS inserter in the filtering angle

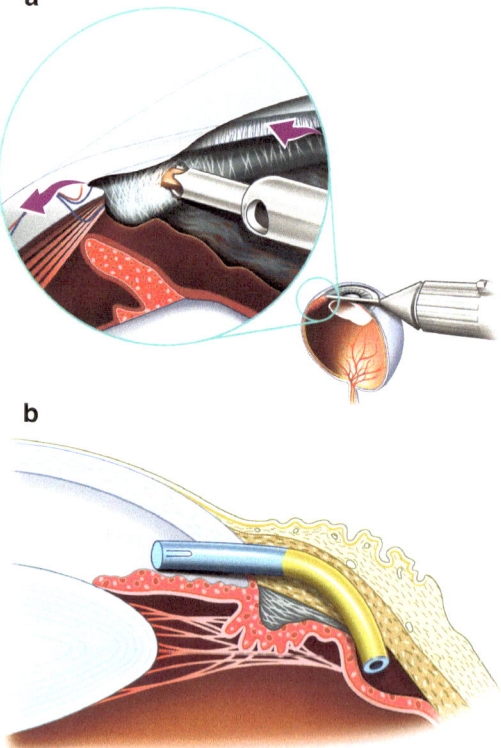

designs and placement alternatives; however all of them are designed to perform the function of enhancing the volume of fluid filtered from the eye.

Typically, once an uneventful phaco procedure is completed, a specially angled mirrored lens (Gonio lens) is placed on the cornea which allows the surgeon to clearly visualize the filtering angle and trabecular meshwork. A handheld delivery system – a "shooter" – is maneuvered into the anterior chamber and across the newly placed lens implant and up against the trabecular meshwork. Once the surgeon is comfortable with the positioning of the operative end of the shooter, they will inject the small stent into the meshwork.

Your job is to confirm that the required materials – the MIGS delivery system, the gonio lens, and an adequate supply of the viscoelastic – are accessible. It is probably prudent to ask your surgeon what materials and ancillary devices he or she might wish to have available on the table. And it is best not to open the stent delivery apparatus until the cataract procedure is successfully completed and your surgeon has confirmed that they are moving ahead with the stent insertion (otherwise you may waste the product).

Chapter 19
Complications Encountered, Instruments at the Ready: Here Is a List of "What-Ifs" and "What to Do's"

Pupil dilation is unsatisfactory for your surgeon:
- Solutions:

    1. Your surgeon may ask for 1% *epinephrine*. This is delivered with a blunt 27-gauge cannula into the AC. Approximately 1 cc is enough. Prior to providing the medication to your surgeon, you should ask the anesthesiologist whether there is any *contraindication* to using this drug within the eye (intra-ocularly). The anesthesiologist may wish to avoid the use of epinephrine in patients with certain cardiac conditions or unstable hypertension.
    2. All else failing, your surgeon may ask for *iris hooks* which are supplied 4–5 to a box and must be handled carefully since they are small and unweidly and may easily end up on the drapes or floor. Pupil expansion rings — of assorted design — are also available to enlarge an undilating pupil.

The surgeon oversizes the wound when manufacturing the main entry, and when attempting to use the phaco tip, too much fluid escapes the eye making for an unstable AC:
- Solution:

    1. Raise the bottle height for more infusion/inflow.
    2. Surgeon to place a 10-0 nylon suture at the end of the wound to shorten its chord length.

The patient is using Flomax©, an oral drug notorious for making the AC unstable and the iris floppy during surgery:
- Solution:

    1. Your surgeon may opt to use *iris hooks or a ring*. Your job would be to supply your surgeon with a toothless *Kelman-McPherson type forceps* to remove each hook from the foam board they are imbedded in. Alternatively, you would perform this function.

© Springer Nature Switzerland AG 2020
R. S. Koplin et al., *The Scrub's Bible*,
https://doi.org/10.1007/978-3-030-44345-0_19

The surgeon will first use a 15-degree angulated blade to make a series of circumferential entries in the peripheral cornea to enter the AC.

Your surgeon will manipulate each hook through the wound to catch the edge of the pupil, then draw the pupil edge toward the corneal wound and then use the small block of plastic at the end of each hook to "lock" the system in place against the cornea.

2. There are several *pupillary ring-like expanders* with inserting mechanisms available on the market. Each one requires special attention and education. Your OR director will in-service you on any available systems.

Your surgeon complains that they are unable to develop adequate aspiration through the IA tip during cortex removal:

• Solution:

1. First check to see that the aspiration line is firmly in place on the handpiece.

   Otherwise, if there was no difficulty with aspiration during the phaco portion of the surgery, the problem is less likely a tubing problem and more likely a blockage in the tip or within the handpiece itself. Remove the handpiece and force saline through it with a 3 cc syringe, and then do the same through the infusion port for the *handpiece*.

   If that does not solve the problem, there may be a blockage in the line, but this is more than likely a function of the cassette/pump. If all else fails, change the cassette.

   The same applies to troubleshooting the phaco portion of procedure; however in this case you must also confirm the stability of the phaco needle. Is it screwed on to the handpiece properly?

The patient exhibits a stark white cataract. This makes performing the capsulorrhexis difficult:

• Solution:

1. *Trypan Blue©* is an innocuous dark blue liquid that is capable of staining the anterior lens capsule when injected into the AC (Fig. 19.1). This makes a world of difference in visualizing the capsule during the capsulotomy. The dye comes

Fig. 19.1 Trypan blue (our stock image)

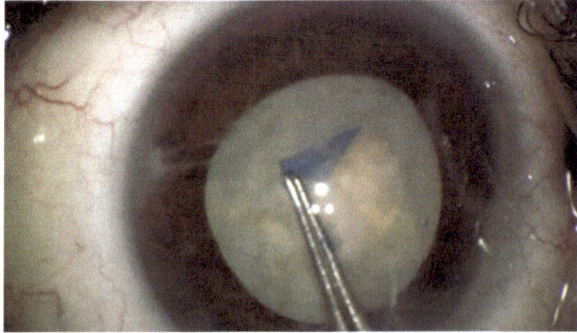

in a syringe not unlike the viscoelastic. You will be required to place a blunt cannula on the syringe.

The process of injection takes place after the incisions in the cornea are made. You will then use a 3 cc syringe with a blunt cannula to simply aspirate air. Hand this to your surgeon (always announce what you are handing over, even if it is obvious). Your surgeon will place a large air bubble in the AC.

You will now hand your surgeon the syringe containing the Trypan Blue©. Your surgeon will paint the anterior capsule with the dye (Fig. 19.1). Following this, you will provide your surgeon with a 3 cc syringe with saline intended to wash the residual Trypan Blue from the AC (perhaps employing the air syringe and filling it with saline). To fill the syringe, remove the plunger and squirt saline from the balanced salt solution container into the shaft. Replace the plunger. Before handing the syringe to your surgeon, purge the syringe of air. To do this, turn the syringe to the upright position and press the plunger slightly, holding your hand over the opening so as not to inadvertently squirt saline around the OR.

Viscoelastic is then used to fill the anterior chamber in preparation of performing the capsulorrhexis.

Your surgeon has noted that the zonules are compromised. Despite this, the surgeon is moving ahead with the phaco surgery:
- Solution:
    - Often, even in the face of zonular pathology, performing the phacoemulsification portion of the procedure can be completed successfully. Hooks, similar to iris hooks, but somewhat longer, can be used to hang over the anterior flap of the capsulotomy in order to stabilize the entire lens-capsular complex. Other techniques to perform the phaco portion of the operation with the lens completely out of the capsular bag may work.
    - Performing the irrigation/aspiration technique, then, becomes the challenge. The I&A aspirates the cortex, which in turn pulls on the capsule, which ultimately stresses the zonules. The danger of disrupting the zonules may lead to multiple complications associated with an unstable lens and presentation of vitreous.
    - The capsular tension ring (CTR) is often used at this stage of the procedure. The CTR is a horseshoe-shaped ring of plastic that is extremely thin and brittle. The ring is compressible which is where it gets its utility, but don't test this since you will likely crack it.
    - The ring is most often supplied *without* an inserter. The inserter is generally available as a reusable metal device which takes some getting used to. The ring segment has eyelets at either end which may be captured by a thin hook that exits as the plunger is depressed on the inserter. Hard to explain, so best to practice on a ring supplied by the manufacturer.
    - The ring is threaded around the inside of the capsular bag. It acts like an expansile spring and will keep the "bag" from collapsing during surgery. It does not cure the deficiency associated with the zonules (the lens may still be

loose), and occasionally, despite a functioning ring, your surgeon may opt to place an IOL elsewhere (rather than in the bag: perhaps in the sulcus or anterior to the iris) or use a suture (10-0 prolene) to capture a haptic and sew it to the iris or fixed to the eye through the sclera (scleral fixation).

Your surgeon announces, perhaps not with the following words, that *the capsule has torn***. This can occur during the phaco portion of the procedure or during the IA; rarely during lens insertion or other maneuvers:**

- Solution:
    - Volumes of academic papers and books have been written about this conundrum. Solomon at his best would not have an answer to every variation on the theme of capsular tears. But here is the short course in what to expect. Depending on your surgeon's personality, temperament, and skill base, there are several choices to consider.
    - Your surgeon's approach will be dictated by the size of the tear (which tends to enlarge during surgery) and the amount of lens material still retained in the various chambers in the eye.
    - Sometimes the nuclear fragments can be removed by opening the main corneal wound a few more millimeters (your surgeon will ask for either the 15 degree or keratome blade), placing a viscoelastic below the lens remnants (attempting to "freeze" them in place) and then using several instruments, such as toothed forceps (Kelman style), and perhaps a micro-spatula, in an attempt to engage and extract nuclear fragments. This is sort of a hand-over-hand technique and is quite arduous. Occasionally, even in the face of a capsular tear, your surgeon will continue the phaco process.
    - The 800-pound gorilla in the room – or in the AC – is the presence of vitreous. This will tend to complicate the issue since the nuclear material – large and small pieces – gets wrapped up in the vitreous making them hard to extricate.
    - At some point, your surgeon may likely call for the vitrectomy handpiece. *Vitrectomy* devices are small cutting systems designed to cut the sticky, gelatinous vitreous, so it can be removed by simultaneous aspiration.
    - To prepare the vitrectomy system, you will simply exchange the phaco handpiece for the vitrectomy handpiece, set the console for vitrectomy, set aspiration and cutting as determined by your surgeon, and run the infusion through the line, ridding the system of air bubbles. If the system is a split device – infusion handpiece and cutting handpiece separate – the tubes will likewise be split between the two instruments.
    - Depending on the elements of complication (i.e., did significant nuclear material escape down the rabbit hole deep into the vitreous cavity, making extraction difficult under the present design of the operation?), the surgeon might ask a retinal specialist to step in (if one was available to complete the vitrectomy and nuclear lens removal). If a retinal specialist is not available, your surgeon will persevere, knowing that the patient will likely need a more complete vitrectomy through a more posterior opening in the sclera on another

day. (This is known as a *pars-plana vitrectomy and would commonly be completed by a retinal specialist*.)

– If the cleanup was successful and appropriate capsule remains available for fixation of a posterior chamber lens, then your surgeon will go forward. If there is insufficient posterior capsule but adequate anterior capsule support, your surgeon may decide to place a PCIOL in the ciliary sulcus in the space between the iris and anterior capsule. Your surgeon will fill this space with viscoelastic and then either inject or fold a three-piece PCIOL into this space. The viscoelastic is then removed with the irrigation and aspiration handpiece.

Following capsule rupture, your surgeon decides the intraocular lens cannot safely be placed in the sulcus:
• Solution:

– Your surgeon may opt to place the lens *in front* of the iris. This requires an anterior chamber intraocular lens.
– Viscoelastic will be used to fill the AC. Your surgeon will ask for the keratome to enlarge the wound (to about 7 mm) and insert the rigid lens (without folding) into the eye over a Sheets Glide, a disposable thin plastic sheet that helps guide the lens into the anterior chamber. Your surgeon will then fashion a hole in the iris (iridectomy) using micro-scissors to prevent fluid blockage. Finally, the viscoelastic will be removed (aspirated with a cannula or the I&A system) and the wound closed with 10-0 nylon sutures (two or more, usually).

• Solution:

– Instead of an anterior chamber lens, your surgeon may decide to suture a posterior chamber lens onto the iris. This requires a three-piece lens with plastic haptics where a prolene suture on a rather long needle (long enough to reach through the cornea, through the iris and back out through the cornea once again) can be looped around the haptic behind the iris and then knotted over the front of the iris.
– Your surgeon will insert the lens using forceps or injector. Miochol may be required to constrict the pupil, trapping the lens optic in position in the AC the haptics are placed *behind* the iris and sutured using 10-0 prolene suture on a long-curved needle. (Circling the suture through the iris and around the haptic is a blind procedure requiring some experience).

• Solution:

– If there is inadequate iris support for suturing a lens, your surgeon may decide to suture or glue a posterior chamber lens into the sclera. Your surgeon will likely request a three-piece PMMA (hard plastic) or foldable lens, both with rigid (PMMA) haptics. Some of these lens styles contain "eyelets," small round circles of plastic at the very end of the rigid haptics, to allow sutures to be attached to them.
– If the lens choice is a solid, PMMA plastic lens, your surgeon will enlarge the corneal wound with a keratome or crescent blade to about 7+ mm.

There are variations in the fixation technique, but generally it involves using 10-0 prolene sutures on a long, curved needle to secure each haptic, through the eyelets, to the sclera. The corneal wound will then be closed with 10-0 nylon sutures. Where a lens haptic is to be glued to an exteriorized pocket in the sclera, there are specific biologic "glues" requested in advance.

During phacoemulsification, the surgeon remarks that the eye is getting firm; concerned, the surgeon may stop the surgery to consider some options. The surgeon may not be sure what is going on:

• Solution:

First the cause of the hard eye needs to be determined:

1. *Choroidal hemorrhage* – this is a rare and potentially devastating complication of any intraocular surgery. Here sudden changes in IOP lead to bleeding from blood vessels in the suprachoroidal space in the back of the eye. As the bleeding continues, the retina and choroid are elevated.

   When this happens, your surgeon may notice a constellation of events. The AC may shallow (as the lens and vitreous move forward in response to the pressure), the eye may become very firm, and there may be a loss of visualization, or a frightening scene as the blood pushes the choroid forward, appearing as a dark mass through the operating microscope. Your surgeon will act very quickly to close the corneal wounds so that the contents of the eye do not get expulsed (pushed out of the eye). Attempts may be made to reform the AC with viscoelastics. In addition, your surgeon may perform posterior sclerotomies (openings in the sclera) to drain suprachoroidal blood from behind the eye.

   Certain characteristics can predispose patients to this condition such as uncontrolled IOP, high myopia, low rigidity of the sclera, high blood pressure, older age, and cardiovascular disease. Abrupt changes in IOP, sudden rise in blood pressure, may trigger this event. The outcome is rarely good.

2. *Aqueous misdirection* – more commonly, the cause of a firm eye in the midst of surgery. In this case there has been a "misdirection" of infused fluids. The saline has slipped behind the lens and is causing an expansion of the vitreous cavity. This in turn pushes the lens/iris diaphragm forward and increases eye pressure. Your surgeon will notice shallowing of the AC and firming of the eye. However, in contrast to choroidal hemorrhage, there will be no loss of the red reflex visible through the operating microscope.

In this case, your surgeon will try to relieve the misdirection. Intravenous drugs may be used including Diamox or mannitol (agents that lower the intraocular pressure). Dilating agents such as atropine may be employed. Your surgeon will fashion a hole in the iris (iridectomy). In some situations, an incision will be made into the pars plana portion of the eye and vitreous aspirated. If the misdirection is relieved, your surgeon may be able to resume the surgery.

Your surgeon notices that the cataract is extremely dense and threatens the security of lens-zonule complex:

- *Solution*:

    Your surgeon decides to convert to an extracapsular cataract extraction instead of proceeding with phacoemulsification (Fig. 19.2). Extracapsular cataract extraction (ECCE) involves the manual removal of the nucleus and was one of the techniques employed for cataract surgery before development of phacoemulsification technology. Although ECCE is an older technique that involves an enlarged wound, it is still used today in cases of overly firm cataracts where the movement of the phaco needle on the cataract may cause complications.

    Your surgeon may plan an extracapsular extraction *prior* to surgery or decide to convert a complicated phacoemulsification to extracapsular surgery *during* the operation.

    Through a small incision (perhaps less than 3 mm), viscoelastic will be placed in the eye and a capsulorrhexis created using a cystitome (or a bent 25G needle) and Utrata-type forceps. Hydrodissection to loosen the nucleus from the cortex will be performed using a 19G cannula with BSS. From this point, the procedure differs from phacoemulsification.

    Your surgeon will enlarge the corneal or scleral wound to 10 mm using a keratome or crescent surgical blade. A singular 7-0 knotted Vicryl suture (synthetic, absorbable, monofilament) will often be placed in the middle of the wound. The surgeon will then need your assitance and hand you the forceps allowing you to hold the cornea aloft while your surgeon extracts the lens.

    Rather than emulsifying the lens, and while you hold the cornea out of harm's way – the nucleus in its entirety is either rotated out of the capsular bag using a pointed instrument such as a cystotome or "expressed" (pushed out), from the capsular bag by gently depressing the inferior limbus with a blunt instrument. This often appears to be rather dramatic as the entire nucleus, often very dark or white in color, exits the eye almost spontaneously through the corneal or scleral wound.

Fig. 19.2 Etracapsular cataract extraction

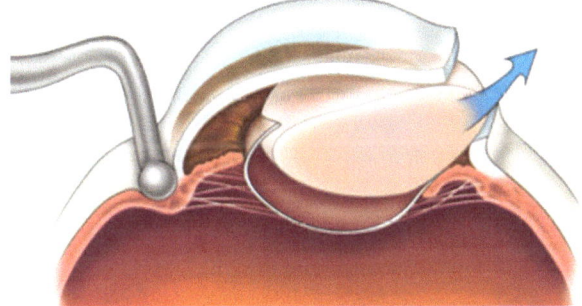

At this point the Vicryl suture is closed, and to either side of this suture, individual 10-0 nylon sutures are placed to further insure a temporary water tight wound as the residual cortex is removed using a standard irrigation and aspiration (IA) handpiece. Once all cortex is removed and the capsule is polished, the capsular bag is examined for defects and if found intact it is inflated with viscoelastic. The central Vicryl suture is removed along with enough 10-0 nylon sutures to permit the insertion of an IOL – usually 7–8 mm. Often your surgeon will insert a three-piece IOL (usually a soft optic portion with firm PMMA haptics). This type of lens is more stable than a single piece IOL.

The lens is placed in the capsular bag if intact or alternatively in front of the bag allowing the haptics to sit in the ciliary sulcus. The viscoelastic is removed and replaced with saline solution. The remainder of the corneal wound will then be closed with 10-0 nylon sutures in order to make a water tight seal.

Chapter 20
The Surgical Tray for Cataract Surgery (Example)

Here you will find the most commonly used instruments in cataract surgery.

The table (tray) – measuring 2 ½ feet by 4 feet – is covered with a plastic backed absorbent sheet.

- Anterior chamber irrigator
- Lid speculums
- 1 keratome (steel or diamond)
- 1 1 degree blade or diamond paracentesis blade
- 1 cystitome
- 1 needle holder
- 1 Kuglen Iris Hook
- 1 Sinskey Hook
- 1 Vannas scissor
- 1 Westcott scissor
- 1 iris spatula
- 1 Utrata-type capsulorrhexis forceps
- Two Tying Forceps: straight and curved
- 1 Kelman style forceps – toothed
- 1 Kelman style forceps – non-toothed
- 1 Colibri forceps
- IOL inserting forceps
- 1 micro-tying forceps straight
- 1 micro-tying forceps curved
- 1 phaco chopper (surgeon's choice)
- Package of mini-cellulose sponges (10) (Weck-Cel (c))
- Sterile cotton swabs (10)
- 1 1 cc syringe + 27 gauge blunt cannula containing 1% lidocaine injectable
- 1 3 cc syringe + blunt 27 gauge cannula filled with BSS
- 1 empty 3 cc syringe (swing)
- 2 27 gauge short needles

© Springer Nature Switzerland AG 2020
R. S. Koplin et al., *The Scrub's Bible*,
https://doi.org/10.1007/978-3-030-44345-0_20

- 1 vial of viscoelastic
- 1 50 cc bottle of sterile balanced salt solution (BSS). (This can be supplied as a factory prepared bottle or as sterile squeeze bottle that can be filled multiple times from protected, capped, bottles of IV saline)
- Phaco parts kit; including wrench and extra silicone sleeves for the phaco and I&A tips. The I&A hand piece will sit here until called for.
- IOL injector (lens implant to be provided at appropriate time)
- Surgeon's gloves
- Surgeon's gown
- Disposable identification stickers to be applied to various injectables

Chapter 21
Surgeon-Specific Instruments

Here are instruments that are personalized depending on the surgeon's unique surgical technique. This is not intended to be an exhaustive list of all instrument options but rather an introduction to their functions with some examples provided.

Speculums Metal devices to hold open the lids, either wire type (which springs open) or screw type (which allows surgeon to set the amount of opening) (Fig. 21.1).

Capsule forceps Forceps with teeth perpendicular to the body of the instrument to allow grasping of the capsule during capsulorrhexis (Fig. 21.2).

Choppers Instruments with a sharp edge either at the side (horizontal chopper) or at the tip (vertical chopper) that allow the surgeon to manually disassemble the nucleus in order to lessen the amount of phaco ultrasound needed (Fig. 21.3).

Lens rotators Instruments with typically a spatula or round end used to rotate the lens (Fig. 21.4).

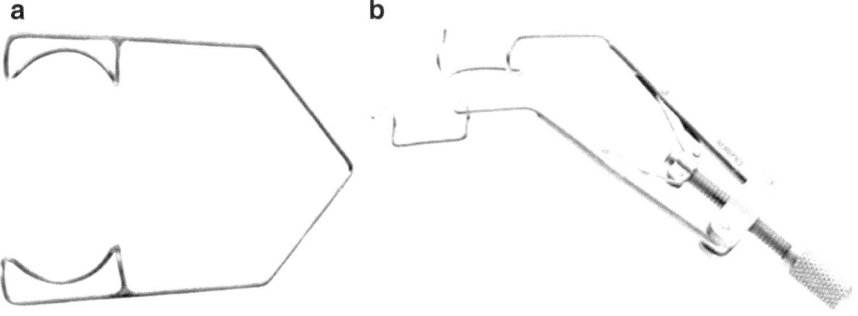

Fig. 21.1 (**a**) Barraquer speculum (**b**) Lieberman speculum. (Courtesy of Katena instruments)

© Springer Nature Switzerland AG 2020   117
R. S. Koplin et al., *The Scrub's Bible*,
https://doi.org/10.1007/978-3-030-44345-0_21

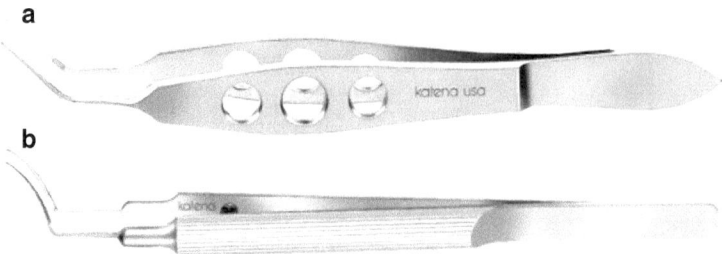

Fig. 21.2 (**a**) Utrata (**b**) Masket. (Courtesy of Katena instruments)

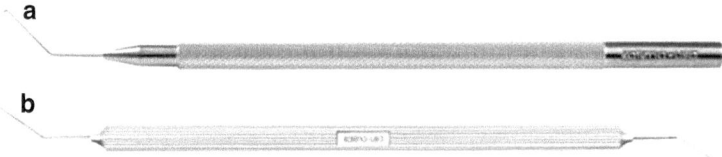

Fig. 21.3 (**a**) Nagahara (**b**) Chang. (Courtesy of Katena instruments)

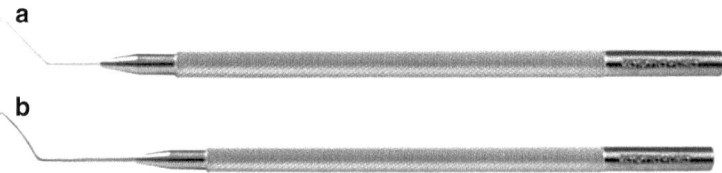

Fig. 21.4 (**a**) Drsydale (**b**) Tennant. (Courtesy of Katena instruments)

IOL manipulators Instruments with a hook at the end to facilitate rotating the intraocular lens into the capsular bag (Fig. 21.5).

Capsule polishers Instruments with a textured surface at the tip, either with sandblasting or coated with carbide diamond to gently abrade and remove residual cortex from posterior capsule (Fig. 21.6).

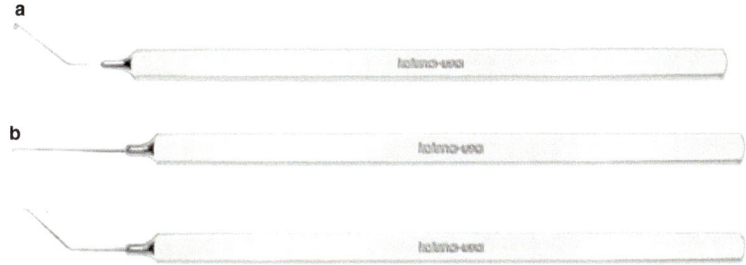

Fig. 21.5 (**a**) Kuglen (**b**) Sinskey. (Courtesy of Katena instruments)

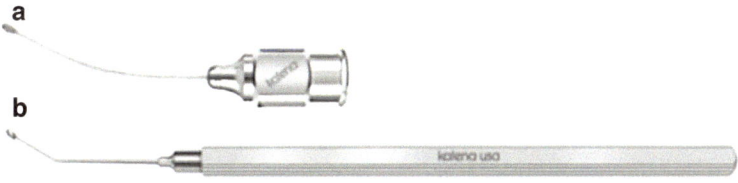

Fig. 21.6 (**a**) Jensen (**b**) Shepherd. (Courtesy of Katena instruments)

Fig. 21.7 Iris hooks.
(Courtesy of Katena
instruments)

Iris hooks, expanders, dilators Devices that facilitate pupil dilation by expanding
the iris (Fig. 21.7).

Toric axis markers Devices used to place orientation marks on the corneal for
implantation of astigmatism correcting lens (Fig. 21.8).

Fig. 21.8 (**a**) Lindstrom
(**b**) Mendez toric marker.
(Courtesy of Katena
instruments)

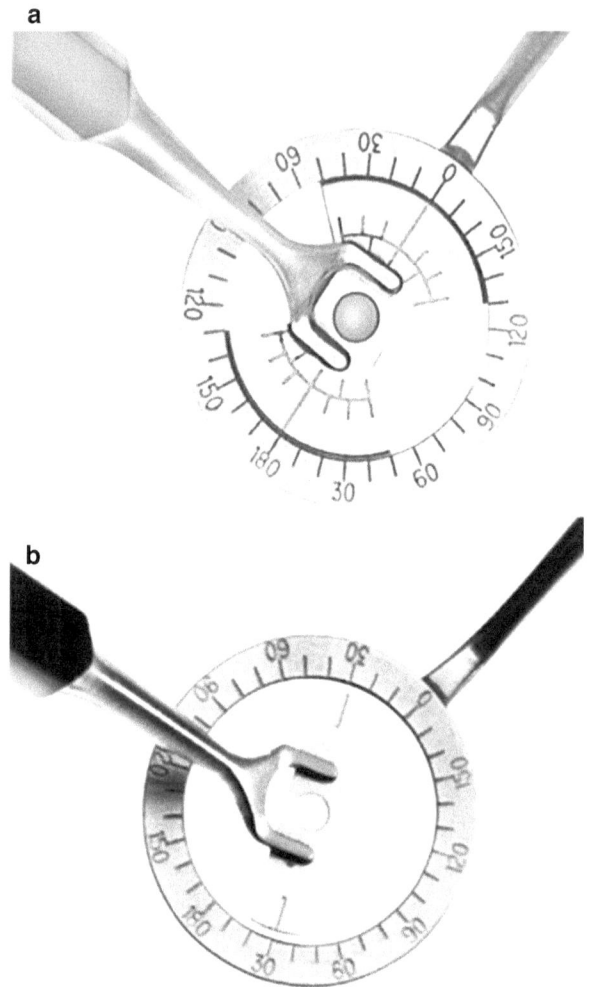

Chapter 22
Self-Assessment Test Cataract Surgery

1. True or False: Modern cataract surgery is minimally invasive. This means that there are virtually no risks to undergoing modern cataract surgery.

   Answer: False. Although modern cataract surgery has reached a unique level of safety and efficacy, no patient should undergo a procedure without understanding the process of informed consent which includes both the rewards and risks to surgery.

2. True or False: The success of an ambulatory surgery center's operations depends on avoiding the stiff state and federal regulations imposed on hospitals. Although the risk to a patient is only minimally greater than a hospital procedure, the cost savings far outweigh this risk.

   Answer: False. An ASC must meet the same standards of care required of a hospital (according to federal, state and local regulations as well as accreditation organizations). Money saving devices are secondary and are never considered where patient safety is in question.

3. True or False: The pupil is actually an opening in the center of the iris, and the lens (cataract) sits behind it.

   Answer: True.

4. True or False: The nucleus is a portion of the lens that makes up its outer portion and is usually quite soft.

   Answer: False. The nucleus is *the inner portion* of the lens and is usually quite a bit firmer than the outer *cortical* portion of the cataract. The nucleus is the portion of the lens that actually undergoes ultrasonic emulsification.

© Springer Nature Switzerland AG 2020
R. S. Koplin et al., *The Scrub's Bible*,
https://doi.org/10.1007/978-3-030-44345-0_22

Fig. 22.1 SuperScrub
sitting on a chair reading
the Iliad in Latin

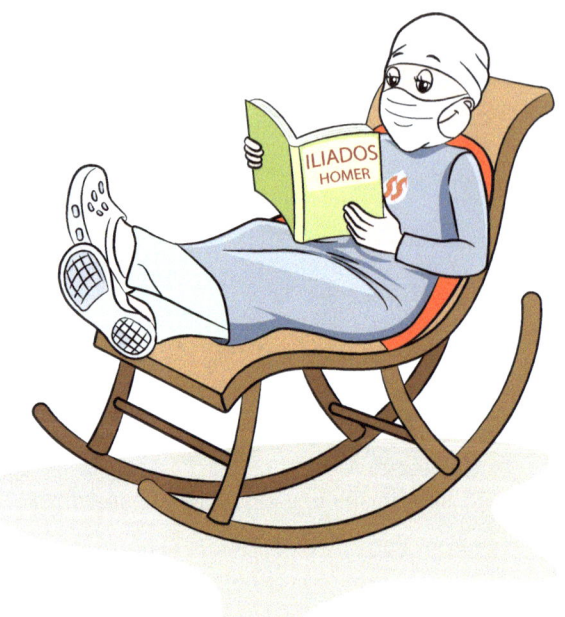

Fig. 22.1 SuperScrub sitting on a chair reading the Iliad in Latin

5. True or False: The cortex is that portion of the lens removed with the irrigation-aspiration handpiece.

   Answer: True. The cortex is soft and therefore does not need emulsification. (The nucleus is removed with the phacoemulsification handpiece.)

6. True or False: Phacoemulsification means "laser-surgery" in Latin.

   Answer: False. Phaco means lens and emulsification means essentially to turn something into "soup." As an aside, often patients mistakenly believe they are having cataract surgery with a laser device.

   Figure 22.1 shows SuperScrub sitting on a chair reading the Iliad in Latin.

7. The single most important objective during the cataract surgery is:

   (a) Strict adherence to the sterile technique
   (b) Completing the operation as quickly and efficiently as possible so as not to invite infection
   (c) Avoiding costly materials that do little to improve outcomes

   Answer: (a) Strict adherence to the sterile technique.

8. Infection control includes:

   (a) Changing into new scrubs when you leave and then return to the ASC
   (b) Performing the first scrub of the day with water and detergent with attention to under-nail areas

(c) Immediately changing gloves when contact is made with a non-sterile object

Answer: All of the above.

9. Proper instrument handling includes:

   (a) Washing instruments one at a time
   (b) Gently but adequately removing any detritus from instruments after surgery in order to avoid baking on materials following sterilization
   (c) Examining instruments for damage prior to sterilization. (Preferably with a microscope stationed in the sterilization room.)
   (d) Flushing any tubular instrument – such phaco-handpieces – forcefully with warm water to remove any debris

   Answer: All of the above.

10. True or False: If you notice a bent instrument on your tray at the time of surgery, it's not necessary to replace it. You might try to fix it yourself by bending it back in shape.

    Answer: False. Any broken instrument should be removed from the OR with a notation to send it for repair.

11. True or False: Since the patient knows which of the two eyes is to be operated upon, verification of the eye to be operated upon is required only of the nursing staff in the preoperative holding area.

    Answer: False. Verification of the operative eye is performed repeatedly prior to the operation and involves notation both written and verbally by the nursing staff, the anesthesiologist, as well as the surgeon both in the preoperative holding area and in the operating suite to confirm the eye, the lens type, and power to be used by your surgeon.

12. True or False: If you do so quietly, it is alright to speak jokingly with your colleagues in the presence of a patient being prepped for surgery.

    Answer: False. Never joke or make whispered comments in the presence of a patient. The patient may take offense or even misconstrue bits and pieces of your conversation.

13. True or False: A *Time Out* is an interruption to the surgery called by the surgeon when a complication occurs.

    Answer: False. A time out is called in the presence of the surgeon, scrub nurse, anesthesiologist, and any circulators at the point of draping the patient and is meant to make final confirmation that the patient is correctly identified, the eye to be operated upon is reconfirmed with a mark over the brow, lens model and power to be used is examined and confirmed, and anesthesia risk is assessed.

14. During surgery, you observe – unbeknownst to the surgeon – that the surgeon's gloved hand brushed a non-sterile portion of the operating microscope. You are concerned about interrupting the surgery. What should you do?

    (a) Call out loudly "unsterile, unsterile," so that everyone in the OR is aware of the danger.
    (b) If it is just the tip of the glove you can probably let it go and avoid the fuss.
    (c) Immediately, and respectfully, make the surgeon aware that there is a lapse in the sterile technique and address the need to change the offended glove before resuming surgery.

    Answer: (c) Your surgeon will appreciate your attention and adherence to the sterile process.

15. True or False: A miotic pupil describes a pupil that is wide open and is important to the success of a cataract procedure.

    Answer: False. A wide pupil is important to facilitate cataract surgery and in this case is in a state of mydriasis or dilation. Miosis refers to a constricted (small) pupil.

16. Which of these instruments is used to perform a capsulotomy?

    (a) A Kuglen Hook
    (b) A nucleus chopping instrument
    (c) A cystitome

    Answer: (c) A cystitome is essentially a bent needle (usually graded 25 gauge) that is bent to accommodate entry into the eye through a small wound.

17. Which of these instruments might be used to continue the flap development to make a continuous curvilinear capsulorrhexis (CCC) once the tear is made by the cystotome?

    (a) Westcott scissors
    (b) Infusion cannula
    (c) Utrata forceps

    Answer: (c) Utrata forceps is designed to grasp the fine edge of the capsulorrhexis and drag it in circumferential pattern.

18. True or False. Air in the tubing of either the phaco or irrigation-aspiration hand-pieces will rarely cause issues to the surgeon during the surgery because the instrument recognizes the bubbles and automatically vents them.

    Answer: False. Air that travels down the tubing will eventually enter the anterior chamber of the eye and obscure the surgeon's visibility. The surgeon will be required to aspirate the bubbles with the handpiece since there is no automatic process to do this.

19. True or False: A viscoelastic is a gel-like substance used by cataract surgeons to fill spaces, such as keeping the anterior chamber formed during capsulorrhexis.

    Answer: True. Viscoelastic substances are very handy, and your surgeon will often use them to safely make maneuvers where fluids will not keep the eye well formed. As example, placing the lens implant in the eye is routinely performed under viscoelastic.

20. True or False: A satisfactory experience for the patient during surgery depends entirely on the skills of the surgeon and how well he/she attends to the complexity of the case at hand.

    Answer: False. The patient – as well as the surgeon – will appreciate a well organized and efficiently run operating room. Often on the first postoperative day, a patient will mention how smoothly things had gone at surgery. Much of the applause, however, should be directed to the Scrub and the OR staff and is a direct reflection of how well prepared they were for the surgery.

21. True or False: Being taught about the advances in cataract surgery is mainly the responsibility of the surgeon who should shepherd you along. Advanced functions in the OR are too complex for you to learn on your own.

    Answer: False. There is nothing about modern cataract surgery that you cannot learn with the assistance of technical manuals, in service sessions, and by paying attention to details. Be "invested" in each procedure being performed and you will become a SuperScrub!

Chapter 23
Surgical Checklist

Preoperative holding area:

√ Did you verify patient allergies?
√ Does the anesthesiologist have any concerns?
√ Did you verify operative eye?
√ Did the surgeon mark the operative eye?
√ Is the pupil dilated adequately (if you believe not, inform the surgeon immediately)

Operating room:

√ Are the microscope and phaco foot pedals properly positioned?
√ Is the patient placed comfortably on the operating table?
√ Is the patient information sheet posted in clear view for the surgeon?
√ Is the intraocular lens available and checked against the surgeon's lens list?
√ Do you have ready surgeon specific instruments?
√ Was a time-out performed?

Typical sequence for an uncomplicated phacoemulsification surgery:

1. Side port incision created.
2. Instillation of anesthetic into the anterior chamber followed by viscoelastic (possible combination of dilation and anesthetic used).
3. Manufacture main operative wound.
4. Inject OVD.
5. Capsulorrhexis (if iris hooks or ring required, they would be placed prior to CCC).
6. Hydrodissection/hydrodelineation.
7. Nucleus fragmentation (cracking or carousel variations) using console setting.
8. Removal of fragment of nuclear lens using console setting.
9. Epinucleus lens material removed using console setting.
10. Cortex removal using irrigation and aspiration handpiece.

© Springer Nature Switzerland AG 2020
R. S. Koplin et al., *The Scrub's Bible*,
https://doi.org/10.1007/978-3-030-44345-0_23

11. Polish capsule.
12. Inflate capsular bag with OVD.
13. Insertion of IOL and positioned.
14. Use I&A for removal of OVD.
15. Wounds hydrated with 25G needle on 3 cc syringe. Wounds checked: suture needed?
16. Topical medications including steroid, NSAID, and antibiotic applied to eye. (Or variation of this theme).
17. Shield/patching of the eye.

    Variations of above are myriad

Chapter 24
Secondary IOLs

Background-Secondary IOLs

There are a multitude of reasons for removing or exchanging an intraocular lens (IOL) after it's been implanted in the eye. These include cases of intraocular lens (IOL) dislocation or subluxation, incorrect lens power, patient dissatisfaction or intolerance, or complications secondary to the lens position, such as inflammation or glaucoma. Once the lens is removed, the patient can be left without a lens (aphakia), or more commonly a secondary IOL can be implanted. Surgical decisions are often based on the clinical presentation, the surgeon's experience, the type of IOL to be used, and the coexisting ocular pathology. A variety of surgical approaches can be used to fixate IOLs outside of the capsular bag including open loop anterior chamber IOL (ACIOL) insertion, iris-claw ACIOL insertion, and posterior chamber IOL (PCIOL) insertion using iris fixation or scleral fixation techniques.

Anesthesia and Patient Preparation

Most surgeons will perform a retrobulbar block (See Chap. 10). Surgeons will vary on position preference. Some prefer to sit at the top of patient's head, others at the temporal position. Ask your surgeon which they prefer so that the microscope and pedals can be set up in the proper orientation.

General Principles and IOL Exchange

The ease of removing an IOL from the eye is dependent on the time since implantation, the amount of scar tissue and fibrosis that encapsulates the haptics, and the location and technique of the initial lens implantation. Removal is easiest if the

© Springer Nature Switzerland AG 2020
R. S. Koplin et al., *The Scrub's Bible*,
https://doi.org/10.1007/978-3-030-44345-0_24

initial implantation was recent, and the lens was implanted without complication into an intact capsular bag and if no posterior capsulotomy has been performed. However, the procedure becomes more complicated if significant time has passed, if there is significant fibrosis of the haptics, or if the capsular integrity is compromised. Generally, the eye volume is increased to stabilize the anterior chamber using an anterior chamber maintainer or with posterior infusion through a pars plana infusion port. You may set up the maintainer using IV pole and tubing with a 23 gauge anterior chamber maintainer or straight from the phacoemulsification machine. If a retinal surgeon is involved, pars plana infusion will be used through one of the sclerotomy ports. Viscoelastic, (typically a cohesive agent like Healon®), is used to viscodissect the capsule from the lens and to free up the haptics from the capsule. Your surgeon may ask for a 30 gauge needle attached to the Healon® cannula which facilitates placing the viscoelastic between the anterior capsular leaflet and the IOL optic. A Kuglen Hook is used to bring the lens out of the bag and anterior to the iris. Depending on the material with which the lens is made, it is either cut in half (Acrylic and Silicone IOL's) with a IOL cutter such as a MST Packer/ Chang IOL cutter, which can fit through a paracentesis incision. A microforceps Alcon 25gauge Grieshaber Revolution® forceps (Figs. 24.1 and 24.2) or MST 23 gauge MST-Microholding forceps is used for countertraction. If the IOL is made of rigid PMMA, it will need to be removed en bloc through a larger corneal wound. Sometimes, surgeons will ask for a Sheets Glide to slip posterior to the IOL so that it does not fall into the back of the eye. Care must be taken to minimize trauma to

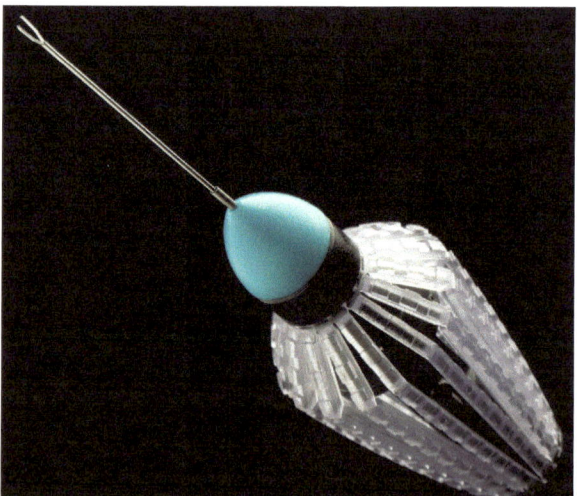

Fig. 24.1 Grieshaber Revolution™ Forceps. (Courtesy of Alcon Labs)

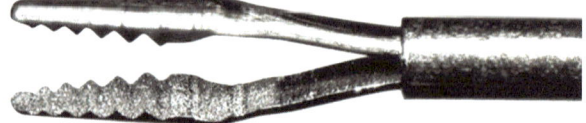

Fig. 24.2 Grieshaber Revolution™ Forceps Tips Closeup. (Courtesy of Alcon Labs)

the endothelial cells that line the cornea when cutting and removing the intraocular lens. If the lens is in the ciliary sulcus, if there is vitreous present in the anterior chamber, or if there is fear of dropping the IOL into the posterior chamber, a retina surgeon is typically present to perform a pars plana vitrectomy and to help bring the lens into the anterior segment.

Secondary Implantation

ACIOL Placement

Some surgeons prefer anterior chamber placement of a new IOL because of its simplicity. The anterior chamber lens (Fig. 24.3) is a rigid style lens usually made of PMMA material and is delivered through a scleral tunnel or a large clear corneal incision. It is then placed flush with the iris so that the haptics are in the "angle" of the eye (where the iris meets the cornea). To prevent pupillary block, or a spike in the intraocular pressure due to mechanical blockage of the aqueous flow, a peripheral iridotomy is typically performed by creating a hole in the peripheral iris using

Fig. 24.3 Anterior chamber IOL. (Courtesy of Alcon Labs)

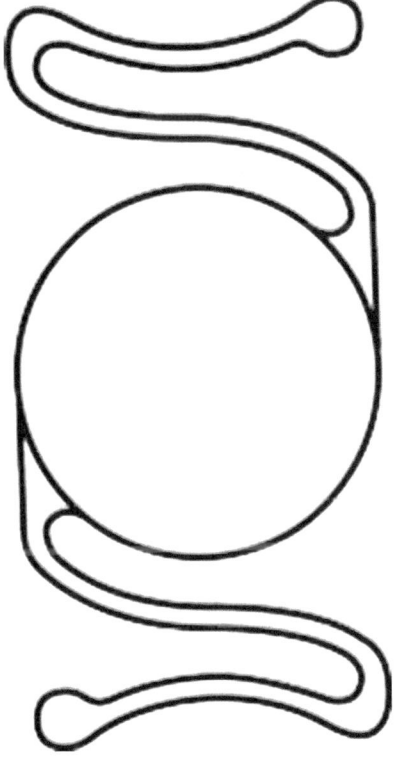

either intraocular scissors or an iris pulling technique. ACIOL placement should only be used in eyes with normal anterior segment architecture, in eyes without significant peripheral anterior synechiae, or low density of endothelial cells.

Surgical Tray IOL Exchange with ACIOL

Instruments
1. Diamond keratome blade (Katena 6579) (Fig. 24.4a)
2. Metal 2.75 mm keratome (Fig. 24.4b)
3. Kuglen Hook (Katena) (Fig. 24.5)
4. Viscoelastic
5. Kelman forceps (Fig. 24.6a, b)
6. 27 or 30 gauge cannulas (Beaver Visitec International)
7. 3 cc syringe
8. Donnenfeld Micro Soft IOL Cutter (Fig. 24.7) or MST Packer/Chang Scissors (MST)
9. Alcon Grieshaber Revolution Forceps or MST-Microholding forceps (MST)
10. Fine needle holder (Katena) (Fig. 24.8)
11. BSS bottle

Fig. 24.4 (**a**) Diamond keratome. (Courtesy Katena Instruments) (**b**) metal keratome (Courtesy Bausch and Lomb)

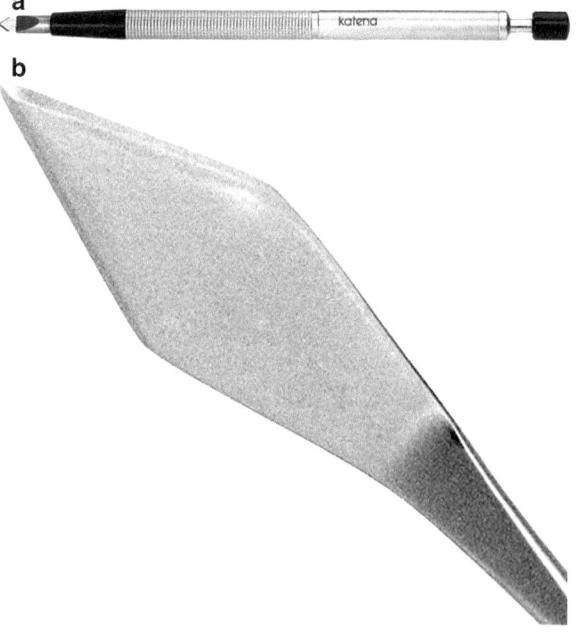

Fig. 24.5 Kuglen Hook. (Katena)

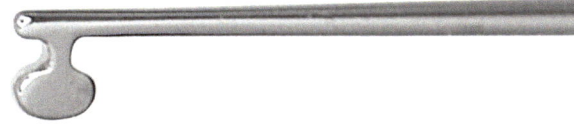

Fig. 24.6 (**a**). Kelman forceps. (Courtesy Katena Instruments). (**b**) Magnified of Tips (Katena)

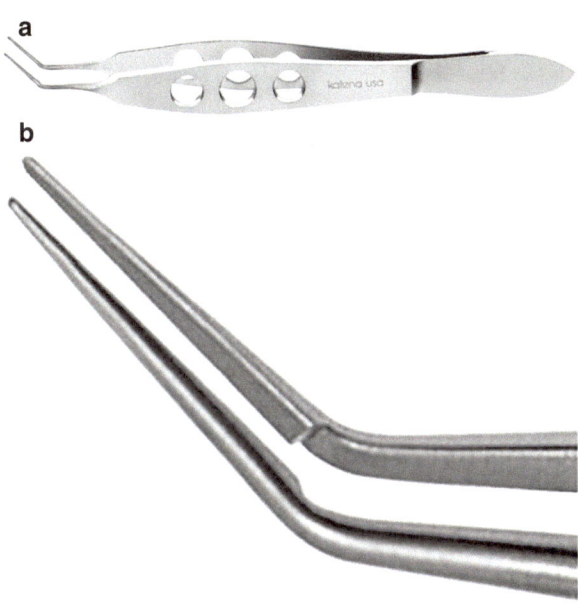

Fig. 24.7 (**a, b**) Donnenfeld Micro Soft IOL Cutter. (Courtesy Katena Instruments) & Mag view

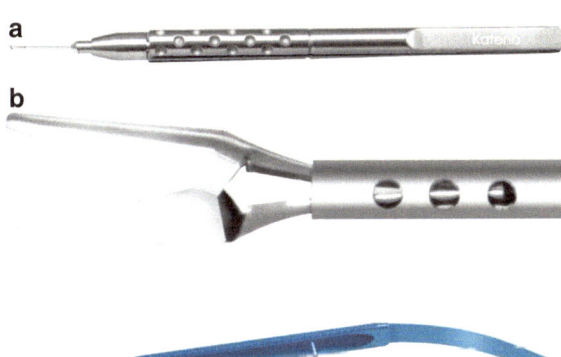

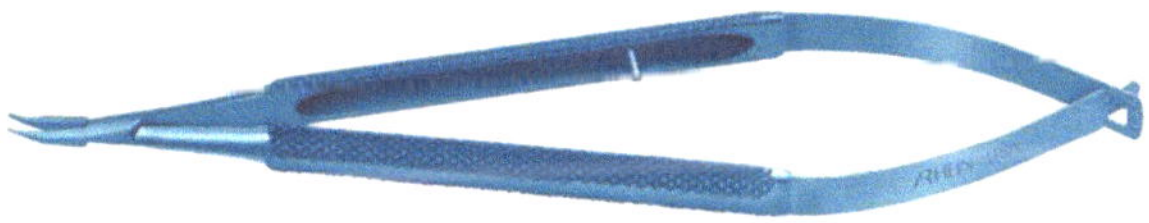

Fig. 24.8 Titanium fine needle holder. (Courtesy Katena Instruments)

Fig. 24.9 Katena
Girard Forceps

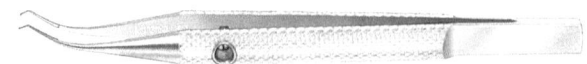

Sutures:
1. 10-0 nylon (Ethicon 160–6 needle or Alcon CU-5 needle)

IOL:
1. Kelman style ACIOL (anterior chamber lenses) MTA2-A5U(12.0–14.5 mm)

Additional:
1. Sheets Glide BD (Beaver Visitec International)
2. Anterior vitrectomy setup

Figure 24.9 Girard forceps.

Secondary Iris Fixation General Principles

Iris fixation is preferable when there is inadequate zonular support or capsular integrity, when the iris architecture is normal, and when there is no history of uveitis or inflammation in the eye. The procedure is relatively quick and minimally traumatic for the patient.

However, some studies show limited shelf-life of the suture material, and the procedure may be complicated by late lens slippage or subluxation postoperatively. To fixate the new lens to the iris, a three-piece lens must be used. The concept of iris suture fixation for posterior chamber intraocular lenses (PCIOLs) dates back to 1976, when Malcolm McCannel, MD, described a transcorneal, retrievable suture technique to refix, resuture, or stabilize subluxated PCIOLs. The modernized version of the technique involves inserting a three-piece, foldable acrylic lens through a 3.25 mm incision and then securing it with a 9-0 or 10-0 Prolene suture. Traditionally the IOL is folded in a mustache technique so that the IOL optic is captured by the pupil, while the haptics extend outward behind the iris. The temporary optic capture stabilizes the lens, while the surgeon places the McCannel iris fixation sutures of both haptics, capturing the free ends through a paracentesis adjacent to the haptic that was captured by the suture. Finally the IOL optic is carefully prolapsed through the pupil to lie behind the iris. The wound is closed with 10-0 nylon sutures (Alcon CU-5 or Ethicon 160–6). Some surgeons place the IOL in an injector and inject the lead haptic under the peripheral iris and rest the optic into the anterior chamber while leaving the trail haptic out of the eye to prevent the IOL from falling into the vitreous. The inferior haptic is then sutured using a McCannel suture technique. The optic is then grasped with the left hand using the microforceps. The optic is pulled anteriorly with the forceps to reveal the outline of the haptic through the iris. Then a 9-0 or 10-0 Prolene suture needle is passed through

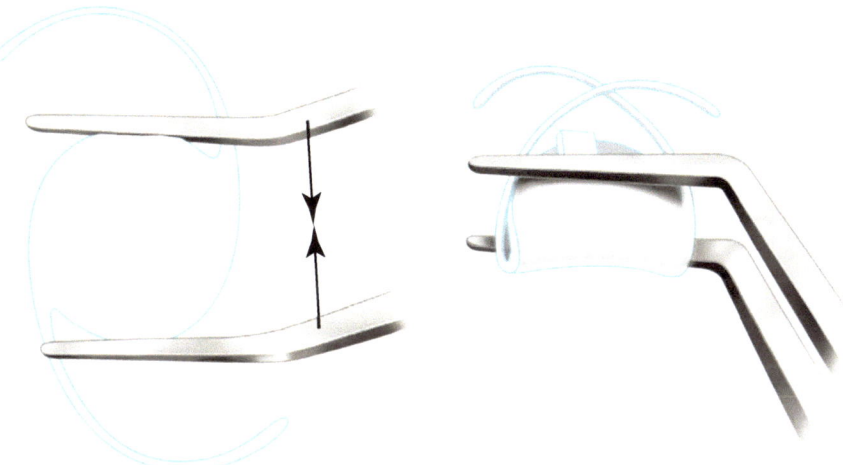

Fig. 24.10 Diagram of mustache fold of IOL

clear cornea through the iris, under the haptic, and then up again through the clear cornea. The needles are removed. A Kuglen Hook is then used to pull the ends of the Prolene suture out of a preplaced paracentesis. The Prolene suture is knotted and placed back through the paracentesis back into the eye thereby fixating the inferior haptics (Fig. 24.10).

Advantages
- Small incision with foldable IOL (3.0–3.5-mm incision)
- Doesn't disturb the conjunctiva (important for eyes with glaucoma)
- Safe in eyes with preexisting superior glaucoma filtering blebs
- No loss of chamber depth
- Minimal induced astigmatism
- Reduced risk of suprachoroidal effusion
- No externalized suture, so reduced risk of endophthalmitis
- Improved suture longevity compared with scleral fixation
- Less challenging than scleral fixation
- May be used perioperatively with cataract surgeries complicated by loss of capsular support during phacoemulsification

Disadvantages
- Requires enough iris tissue to support a lens
- Suturing technique may disturb the shape of the pupil and create "ovaling"
- Potential loss of the IOL into the posterior chamber, if there is less-than-adequate pupillary capture or the suture does not adequately capture a haptic
- Not suited for a silicone lens, which are slippery and difficult to maneuver
- Should not be attempted without significant practice on animal or cadaver eyes

Surgical Tray IOL Exchange with Iris Fixation

Instruments
1. Diamond or metal keratome blade
2. Fine needle holder
3. Kuglen Hook
4. Viscoelastic (Healon™)
5. Kelman forceps
6. 27 or 30 gauge cannula
7. Donnenfeld Micro Soft IOL Cutter or MST Packer/Chang Scissors
8. Alcon 25 g Grieshaber Revolution Forceps or MST-Microholding forceps
9. Girard forceps

Sutures:
1. 10-0 or 9-0 Prolene™(Polypropylene suture) on CTC-6 L,CIF-4, or STC-6 needles (Ethicon) for iris fixation
2. Suture for corneal wound (10-0 nylon Alcon CU-5 or Ethicon 160–6)

Scleral Fixation Techniques

For scleral fixation, the three most commonly performed techniques are scleral sutured, glue-assisted scleral fixation with sclera flaps, and the Yamane flanged IOL technique.

1. Scleral suture fixation (ab interno and ab externo techniques)
2. Sutureless, fibrin glue-assisted PCIOL implantation with intrascleral tunnel fixation or "glued IOL technique"(Agarwal)
3. Sutureless needle-guided intrascleral IOL technique or "Yamane flanged IOL technique."

Early scleral suture fixation techniques involve tying knots directly to the haptic of a one-piece rigid PMMA lens. The Alcon CZ70BD (Fig. 24.11) PMMA lens contains eyelets for such suture fixation. The disadvantage of the use of this lens is the IOL is rigid and the 6.5 mm optic requires a 7 mm incision. Most surgeons have abandoned suturing large diameter PMMA lens.

Ab externo suture fixation (sutures passed from outside eye into the eye)
Ab externo fixation refers to scleral fixation in which sutures are passed from the outside to the inside of the eye. Most surgeons utilize 9-0 or 10-0 double-armed polypropylene suture (Prolene™). The suture needle may be straight (Ethicon™ 10-0 Prolene STC-6), which provides longer range of access, or curved (Ethicon™ 10-0 Prolene CIF-4) or (Ethicon 10-0 Prolene CTC-6), which provides a more rigid curved needle. A hollow 25 or 27 gauge needle can be used as a docking guide to ensure exit of the suture needle through the correct site in the sclera. Scleral flaps, tunnels, or grooves can be used to protect the knot and prevent external suture erosion.

Fig. 24.11 CZ70BD
PMMA IOL. (Courtesy
Alcon Labs)

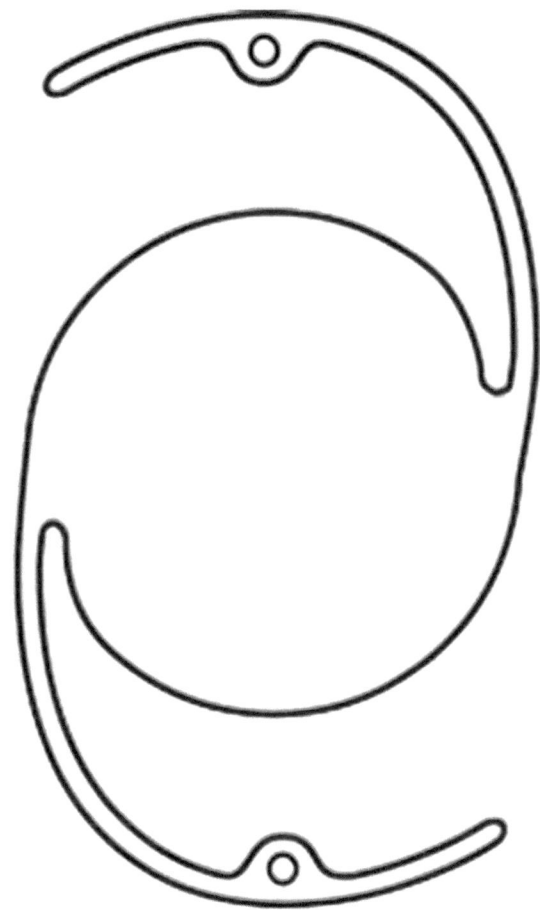

Ab interno suture fixation (sutures passed form inside eye to outside of the eye)

In ab interno fixation, the suture is passed from the inside to the outside of the eye. In order to avoid a blind pass through the ciliary sulcus, the suture needle can be inserted into and externalized using a hollow needle that was placed at a known landmark or by utilizing endoscopic visualization. Recently some authors have been using foldable IOLs including the Bausch & Lomb Akreos AO60 (Fig. 24.12) a hydrophilic acrylic lens contains four eyelets or The Bausch & Lomb enVista® MX60E IOL (Fig. 24.13) that is a hydrophobic acrylic IOL that contains two eyelets. Each lens has a 6 mm optic but will fold and can be placed through a 3.25 mm incision. Most authors prefer fixation with a Gore-Tex CV-8 sutures (equivalent to about 7-0 gauge) with these lenses. They are difficult to bury in anything smaller than a 23 gauge needle whole, and the needle in the GoreTex CV-8 is not as sharp as its Prolene suture counterparts.

Fig. 24.12 Akreos AO60
IOL. (Courtesy Bausch
and Lomb)

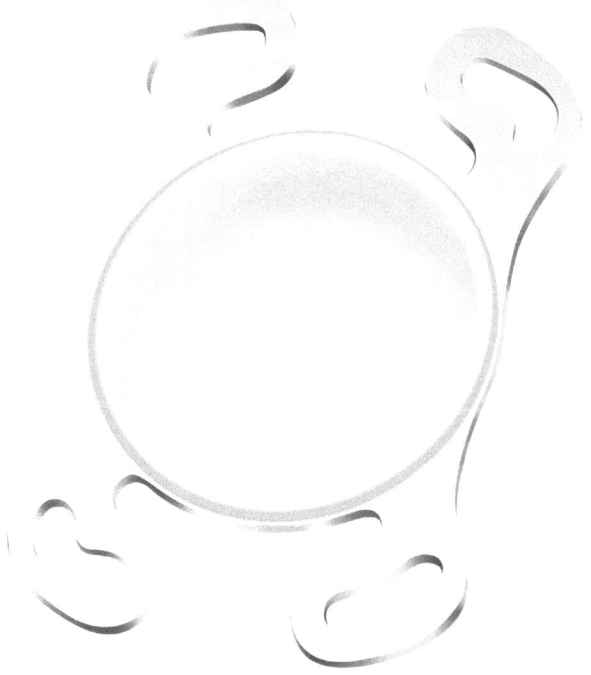

A dislocated IOL capsular bag complex (Fig. 24.14) may also be fixated by passing the suture needle through the capsular bag. The suture can be passed from the
outside to the inside of the eye. Most surgeons use 9-0 or 10-0 double-armed polypropylene suture (Prolene). The needle may be straight (Prolene from Ethicon
STC-6), which provides longer range of access, or curved (Ethicon CIF-4 or
CTC-6). A hollow 27 gauge needle can be used as a docking guide to ensure exit of
the suture needle through the correct site in the sclera. The knot is then buried to
prevent erosion and complications from the knot. Some surgeons prefer the Hoffman
corneal scleral pocket technique that is less likely to be complicated by suture
erosion.

Surgical Tray Scleral Fixation with Sutures

Instruments:
1. Needle holder (titanium fine curved non-locking needle holder)
2. Girard forceps
3. Kuglen Hook
4. 27 gauge hollow needle
5. Metal or diamond keratome
6. Cautery with erasure tip

Fig. 24.13 enVista®
MX60E IOL. (Courtesy
Bausch and Lomb)

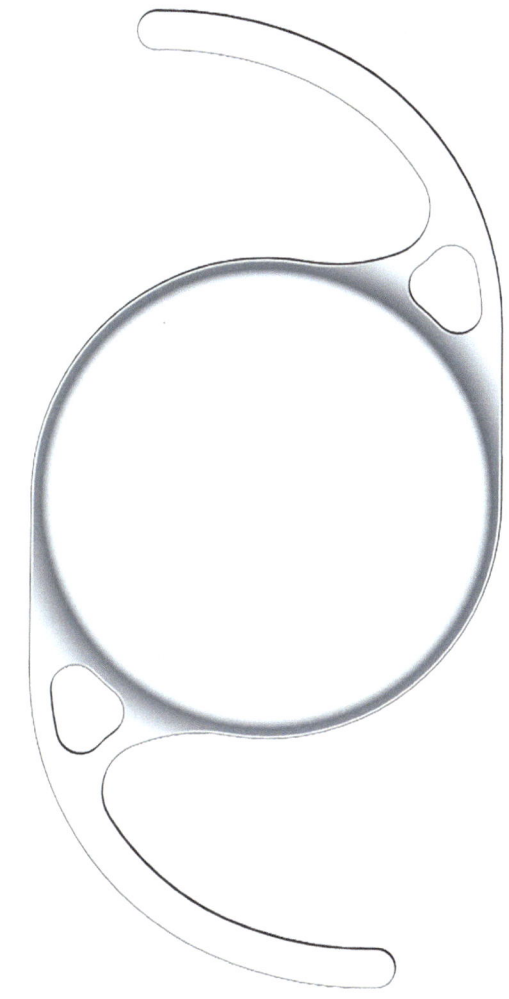

Fig. 24.14 Dislocation
IOL/capsular bag complex
inferiorly. (Our
Stock Image)

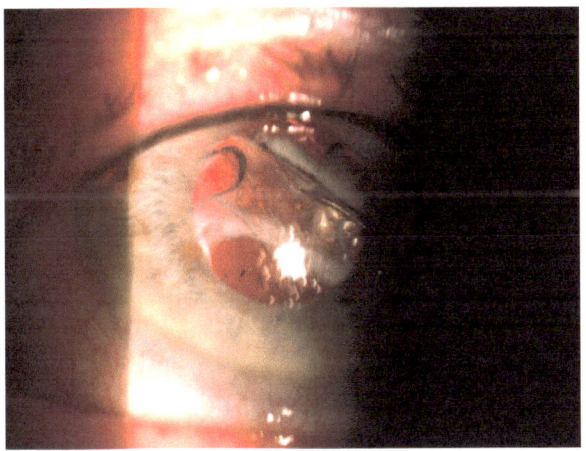

Suture material:
1. Polypropylene (Prolene 9-0 and 10-0 Sutures).
2. Gore-Tex sutures (W.L. Gore & Associates, Elkton, Maryland, USA) is a non-absorbable, polytetrafluoroethylene monofilament suture. Gore-Tex has greater tensile strength and has been reported to have lower suture breakage rates when used in the eye.

IOLs:
1. Rigid PMMA with eyelets (Alcon CZ70BD)
2. Bausch & Lomb Akreos AO60 acrylic lens with four eyelets
3. Bausch & Lomb enVista MX60E acrylic lens with two eyelets

Scleral Fixation Sutureless Techniques

Agarwal Technique: Glue-Assisted Scleral Fixation with Scleral Flaps

For this sutureless scleral fixation technique, the IOL haptics can be externalized and fixated to the sclera without sutures. Typically, a limbal conjunctival peritomy is performed followed by the creation of two partial thickness flaps that are created in the sclera 180 degrees apart using a crescent blade (Fig. 24.15). Wet field cautery is employed for hemostatis. In these meridians, sclerotomies can be created approximately 1.00 mm to 1.50 mm from the limbus using a 20 gauge or 23 gauge micro-vitreoretinal blade. A diamond keratome is used to create a clear corneal incision (3.00 mm to 3.25 mm). If present, the original IOL can be removed en bloc or after cutting with an IOL scissor. If a non-foldable PMMA IOL was present, the corneal incision is enlarged to 6.0 mm to accommodate its removal. A new foldable three-piece acrylic preferably a Zeiss CT-Lucia (Fig. 24.16a, b) is placed in its proprietary injector and injected into the eye where the leading haptic is externalized using a microforceps (25 gauge disposable Grieshaber Revolution forceps or MST endoforceps) through the preplaced sclerotomy. As the optic is passed into the posterior chamber, an additional retinal endoforceps is used to grasp the trailing haptic and externalize it through the second sclerotomy in a "handshake technique." Partial-thickness scleral tunnels are created adjacent to each sclerotomy using a 25 gauge needle with countertraction using a Castroveijo 0.12 forceps (Fig. 24.17). The haptics are then threaded through these tunnels to fixate the IOL. The tunnel direction and depth is adjusted until the optic is centered and there is no appreciable tilt of the IOL. Tisseel™ fibrin adhesive glue is used to close the scleral flaps and the overlying conjunctiva. The corneal incision is closed using 10-0 nylon sutures.

Surgical Tray Glue-Assisted Scleral Fixation with Scleral Flaps
1. Crescent blade
2. Grieshaber Revolution Disposable Forceps (Alcon Labs) or MST endoforceps
3. MVR blade 23 or 21 gauge

Fig. 24.15 Crescent blade.
(Courtesy of Katena
Instruments)

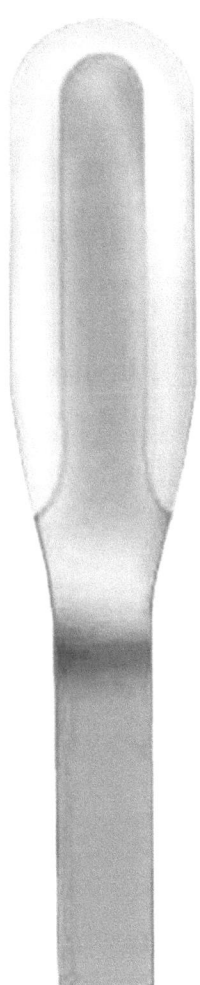

4. Non-locking fine curved needle holder
5. Forceps (Girard or Castroviejo 0.12 forceps)
6. Tisseel Fibrin Sealant (Baxter Healthcare Corporation, Deerfield, IL, USA)
7. 25 or 26 gauge needle for tunnel creation
8. Tennant Tying Forceps (Katena)

IOL
1. Zeiss CT Lucia 602 (formerly EC-3PAL)
2. Tecnis ZA9003 (Johnson and Johnson Vision)
3. MA60MA (Alcon Laboratories)

Sutures
1. 10-0 nylon (Alcon CU-5 or Ethicon 160–6 Needles)

Fig. 24.16 (**a**) CT Lucia
IOL and (**b**) Injector.
(Courtesy of Zeiss)

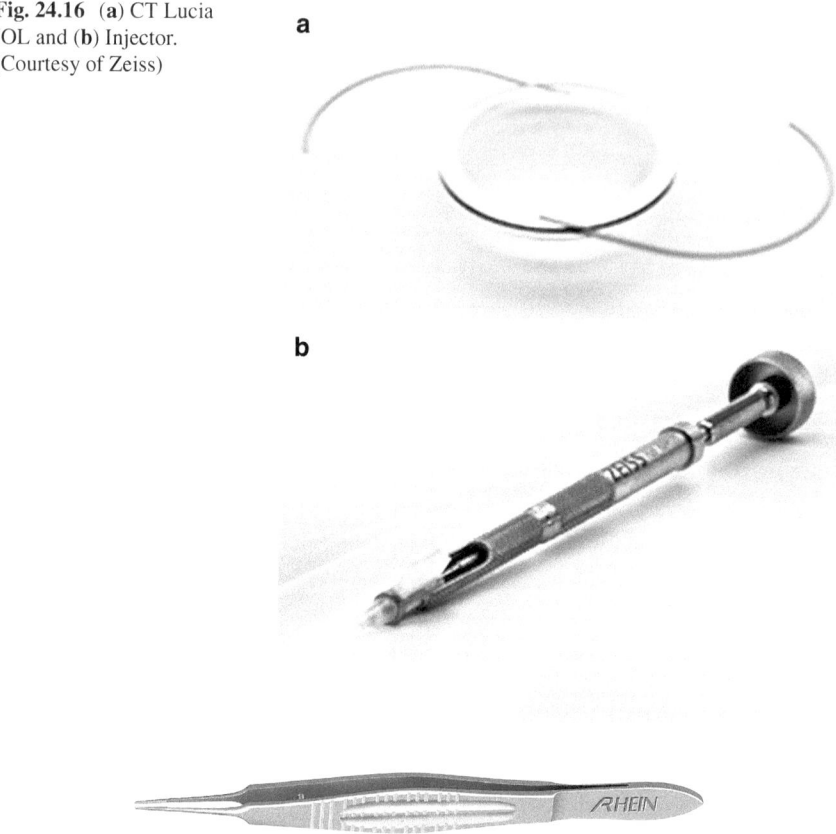

Fig. 24.17 Castroviejo 0.12 forceps. (Courtesy of Katena Instruments)

Infusion
1. AC maintainer connected to BSS on pole
2. Pars plana infusion through sclerotomy

Yamane flanged intraocular lens implantation with lamellar scleral dissection
The sutureless, needle-guided, intrascleral IOL technique was first described by
Shin Yamane MD. It is relatively quick, is sutureless, and is minimally traumatic to
the eye. A toric IOL marker is used to place marks 180 meridians to guide the entry
sites of 30 gauge needles to help align the IOL haptics. A three-piece foldable
acrylic IOL (Zeiss CT Lucia 602) is inserted into the anterior chamber using an
injector, and the trailing haptic is kept outside to prevent the IOL from falling into
the vitreous cavity. An angled sclerotomy is made through the conjunctiva using a
30 gauge thin-walled needle at 2 mm from the limbs (Fig. 24.19). The IOL is placed
into the eye, and the lead haptics is docked into the lumen of a needle and then
threaded into the lumen of the needle using a retinal endoforceps. The needle/haptic
complex is then externalized. The tip of the haptic is cauterized so that a small nub

approximately 0.3 mm is formed which prevents the haptic from slipping back into the eye. A low-temp pinpoint cautery device is used for this procedure. A second sclerotomy then is made with a 30 gauge thin-walled needle that was 180 from the first sclerotomy. The second haptic is then placed through the wound into the eye and threaded into the lumen of the second 30 gauge needle. The second needle and haptic are externalized through the conjunctiva. The surgeon can then estimate how far down the second haptic to cauterize to match the first haptic. The corneal incision is closed using 10-0 nylon sutures. The flange of the haptics are then pushed back and fixed into the scleral tunnels.

Surgical Tray Yamane Technique
1. Diamond keratome or 2.75 mm metal keratome
2. Alcon Grieshaber Revolution Forceps or MST endoforceps
3. Curved fine non locking needle holder (Katena Instruments)
4. Forceps (Girard or Castroviejo 0.12 forceps)
5. TSK ultra-thin-walled needle (Tochigi Seiko, Tochigi, Japan) (Fig. 24.18)
6. Low-temp fine cautery (Accu-Temp Cautery, Beaver Visitec International)
7. Tennant Tying Forceps (straight and curved)-(Katena Instruments) (Fig. 24.19)
8. BSS bottle
9. AC maintainer connected to IV pole with BSS bottle for infusion

Sutures:
1. 10-0 nylon (Alcon CU-5 or Ethicon 160–6)

IOL:
1. Zeiss CT Lucia 602 (Zeiss)
2. Tecnis ZA9003 (Abbott Medical Optics, Santa Ana, CA)
3. MA60MA (Alcon Laboratories)

Fig. 24.18 TSK 30 gauge thin-walled needle. (Our image)

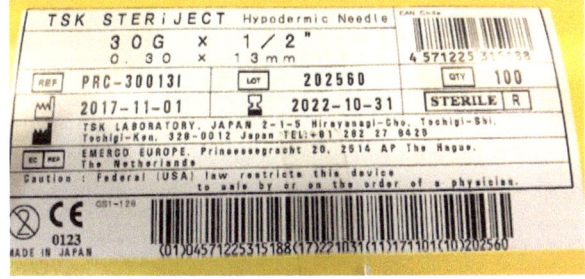

Fig. 24.19 (a, b) Tennant Tying Forceps. (Katena)

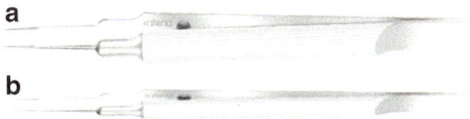

Chapter 25
Corneal Surgery: The Cornea – How It Works

The cornea is the "window" into the eye. It is the transparent tissue that forms the dome in the front part of the eye. The cornea is comprised of three layers (Fig. 25.1). The outer layer, the epithelium, protects against infection, injury, and dryness. The central layer that forms the bulk of the cornea, the stroma, is comprised of fibers that provide strength. The inner layer, the endothelium, consists of cells that actively pump fluid out of the cornea so it maintains transparency. Unlike most other tissues in the body, the cornea is devoid of blood vessels to allow for transparency.

Damage to any of the layers of the cornea can result in swelling or clouding of the cornea, decreasing the corneal transparency. The cornea can lose its clarity from swelling (accumulation of fluid), scarring, perforation, loss of tissue, or development of blood vessels. These processes can occur from many causes, such as trauma, infection, inflammation, and degeneration of the corneal layers. If the cornea becomes opaque, the ability of the eye to see through it is reduced.

Fig. 25.1 Corneal layers

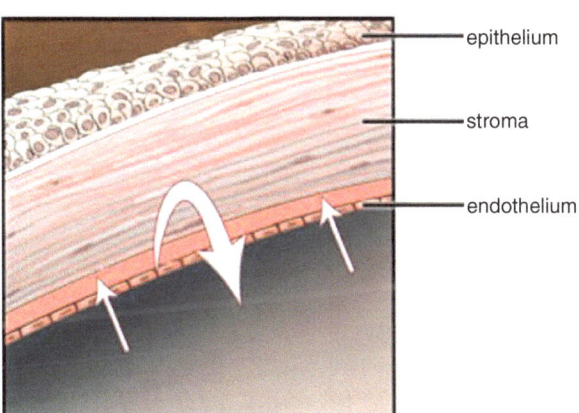

epithelium

stroma

endothelium

© Springer Nature Switzerland AG 2020
R. S. Koplin et al., *The Scrub's Bible*,
https://doi.org/10.1007/978-3-030-44345-0_25

Surgery of the Cornea

Corneal surgery can be technically challenging and is typically performed by surgeons with specialized training in corneal surgery. Corneal surgery refers to any operations that involve the cornea. It encompasses corneal transplants to remove either part of the cornea or the entire cornea, removal of abnormal growths from the surface of the cornea, and reshaping the cornea such as in refractive laser vision correction. Most corneal surgeries are performed in an operating room, with the exception of laser vision correction that can be performed in a laser suite.

Most patients that require corneal surgery are counseled by their surgeons regarding the procedure and length of recovery. For instance, the recovery period after a full thickness corneal transplant to attain good vision is typically prolonged and may take over a year. The risks may also be more involved as the surgery is more invasive than, for example, cataract surgery. Likewise, the surgery itself tends to be more extensive than cataract surgery, requiring more time and instrumentation. Your preparedness and attention to details are vital to the smooth flow of the operation.

Patient Preparation and Anesthesia

Preparing the patient for corneal surgery in the operating room is similar to cataract surgery. Please refer to the earlier section on patient prep. One notable difference is that corneal surgery often requires a longer duration of anesthesia. Your surgeon and anesthesiologist will determine whether the patient requires general anesthesia or monitored anesthesia care (MAC). This will depend on the patient's age, anxiety level, and the complexity of the surgery.

In most cases of corneal surgery, monitored anesthesia care is sufficient. An anesthesiologist or, alternatively, a nurse anesthetist working under the direction of an anesthesiologist will insert an IV, usually in the antecubital fossa (where the elbow bends) or the back of the hand, or forearm. Medications are then delivered via the IV to relax the patient. Agents commonly used include a short-acting opioid analgesic such as a Fentanyl, a benzodiazepine such as midazolam (Versed®), or a hypnotic agent like propofol (Diprivan®). Midazolam and propofol have the additional effect of causing amnesia so that the patient may not remember the procedure. These agents are generally safe in the amount and duration given for eye surgery, though fentanyl can cause nausea, dry mouth, confusion, and weakness and propofol is associated with low blood pressure and transient apnea (suspension of breathing).

In addition to MAC anesthesia, regional anesthesia in the form of retrobulbar block is often done for corneal surgery. *Retrobulbar anesthesia*, which gives the longest duration of regional anesthesia and additionally causes akinesia (lack of eye movement), is given deep in the orbit just outside the cone of extraocular muscles. Because the injection is given deep into the orbit where there are adjacent delicate structures such as the eye, optic nerve, extraocular muscles, and blood vessels, retrobulbar anesthesia in rare cases can cause complications such as eye perforation, irreversible vision loss, permanent double vision, or cardiorespiratory arrest.

After the anesthesiologist or nurse anesthetist has placed the EKG monitors, blood pressure cuff, and started administering MAC sedation through the IV, the retrobulbar anesthetic is given by your surgeon. To prepare this, a 25 gauge needle is used to draw up a mixture of the appropriate anesthetic, typically 50:50 mixture of 2% lidocaine with 0.75% marcaine. Some surgeons prefer adding hyaluronidase that helps the anesthetic to dissolve in the tissue better. Once this is drawn up, a 25 gauge long needle (1.5 inches) or an Atkinson needle, specific for retrobulbar injection, is placed. Your surgeon will then inject the anesthetic into the retrobulbar space and apply mild pressure to the globe with a gauze pad. The remainder of the patient prep, cleaning the eye and draping, is similar to cataract surgery.

Contemplating Corneal Transplant

In the normal eye, the cornea is transparent to allow for clear vision. The clarity of the cornea is maintained by a layer of cells (endothelial cells) that line the back of the cornea and continuously pump fluid out of the cornea. In addition, there are no blood vessels or lymphatic vessels in the cornea. With certain eye diseases (Fig. 25.2), the cornea may become cloudy. This may be due to a variety of problems including swelling, scarring, formation of blood vessels, and thinning or frank perforation of the cornea. Conditions ranging from infection, inflammation, trauma, degeneration, or congenital issues may also degrade corneal clarity.

Often, medical therapy is attempted first. However, when the cornea clouding is irreversible, a corneal transplant may be the only option to restore vision.

Modern corneal transplant surgery is an outpatient procedure, performed either in an ambulatory surgery center or in a hospital. An overnight hospital stay is almost never required other than if the patient is blind in the other eye or if there are social reasons the patient is unable to be cared for following the surgery.

Although corneal transplant surgery may seem daunting to patients, it is relatively straightforward compared to other organ transplants. For instance, there is typically no waitlist or waiting time for cornea tissue. Unlike other organs, the cornea does not need to be matched to the specific recipient, because it is devoid of blood vessels. Therefore, any cornea deemed to be suitable for transplantation can be applied to any patient. Second, concerted efforts by eye banks across the country

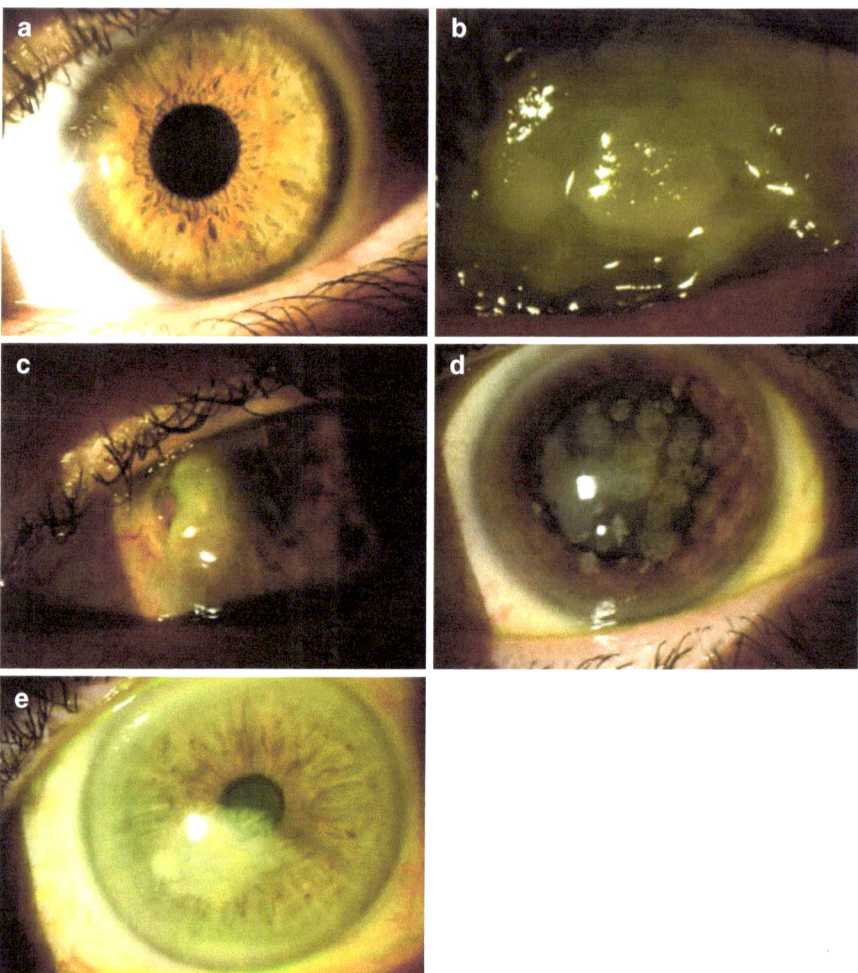

Fig. 25.2 Examples of cornea pathology (**a**) normal cornea, (**b**) cornea ulcer, (**c**) cornea perforation, (**d**) cornea dystrophy, (**e**) cornea scar (Scrubs Bible Version 1)

to recruit donors have resulted in reasonable availability of corneas. Annually, over 45,000 cornea transplantations are performed in the United States.

Figure 25.3 shows SuperScrub carrying a box labeled eye bank: gift of sight.

Your surgeon will have counseled the patient extensively about receiving a corneal transplant. A decision will be made regarding the type of corneal transplant the patient will receive, either a full thickness transplant called penetrating keratoplasty or a partial thickness transplant called an endothelial keratoplasty. Each requires specific instrumentation tailored to the operation.

Fig. 25.3 SuperScrub carrying a box labeled eye bank: gift of sight (Scrubs Bible Version 1)

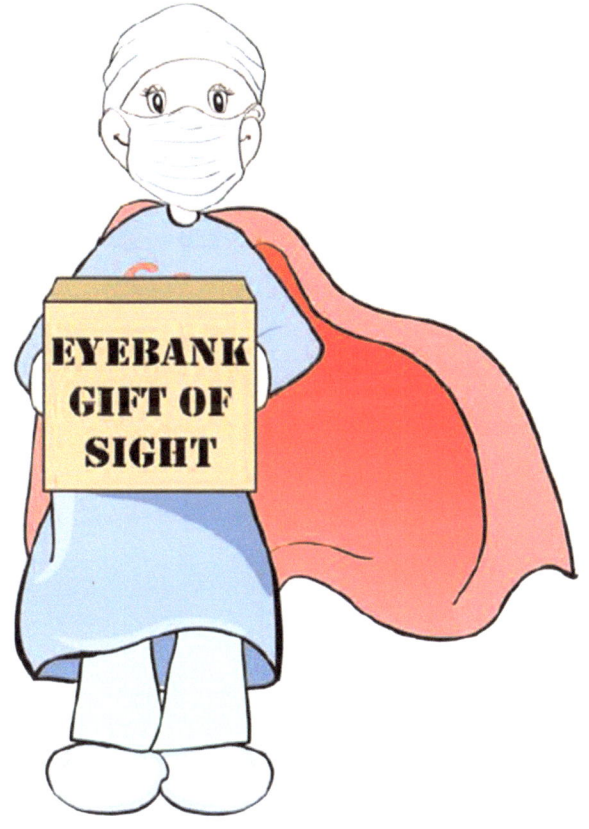

Chapter 26
Corneal Transplantation: Penetrating Keratoplasty

Traditionally, the most common form of corneal transplantation is *penetrating keratoplasty (PK)*. In PK, the entire thickness of the cornea is removed and replaced with a full-thickness donor cornea. This has been the default operation when cornea transplant is deemed necessary, whether it be for corneal swelling, scarring, irregular corneal shape, or perforation. However, with advent of selective replacement of certain layers of the cornea, the reasons for obtaining a full-thickness corneal transplant have become more selective. Indications for a PK include but are not limited to corneal dystrophies and degenerations, congenital or acquired corneal opacities, trauma or scarring from inflammation or infection, and decompensation after cataract surgery not amenable to endothelial keratoplasty.

The Operation

The basic principle of PK is full-thickness removal of patient's cornea and replacement with a donor cornea that is then secured with sutures (Fig. 26.1).

Stabilizing the Eye

Depending on individual preference, some surgeon may stabilize the eye with a Flieringa scleral fixation rings (Fig. 26.2). The Flieringa ring is a stainless steel ring that can be sutured to the sclera. It serves to maintain the structure of the globe once the cornea is removed so that the globe does not collapse onto itself. Your surgeon may utilize the Flieringa ring in all PK cases or only in cases that are at high risk for

© Springer Nature Switzerland AG 2020   151
R. S. Koplin et al., *The Scrub's Bible*,
https://doi.org/10.1007/978-3-030-44345-0_26

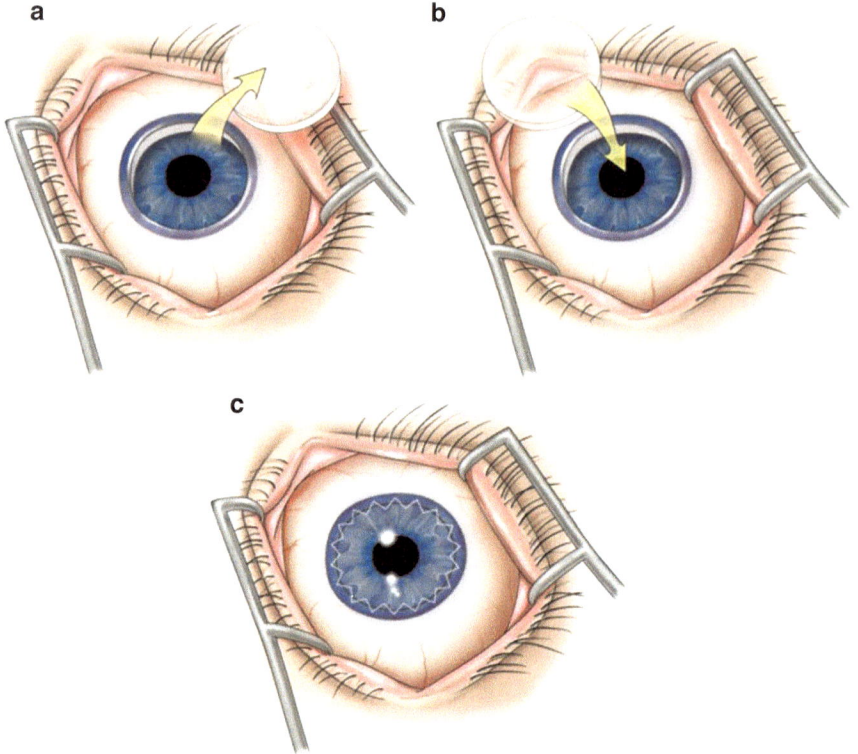

Fig. 26.1 (**a–c**) Penetrating keratoplasty schematic. (**a**) Removal of diseased cornea. (**b**) Replacement with donor cornea. (**c**) Donor cornea secured with sutures

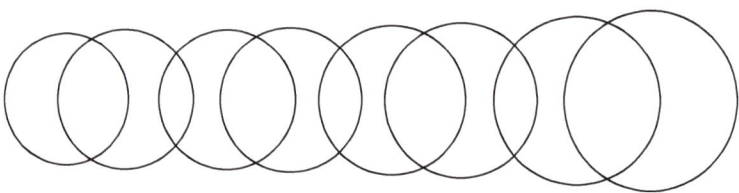

Fig. 26.2 Flieringa rings. (Courtesy of Katena instruments (Scrubs Bible Version 1))

scleral collapse, such as aphakic eyes, pediatric patients, highly myopic eyes, or in eyes that has had prior vitrectomy surgery. The rings come in various sizes. Your surgeon will select an appropriate size based on the patient's cornea diameter and the amount of adnexal exposure. The ring is then sutured to the sclera in four quadrants typically using 7-0 vicryl or 7-0 silk sutures (Fig. 26.3).

Fig. 26.3 Flieringa ring
secured on to eye. (Our
stock image)

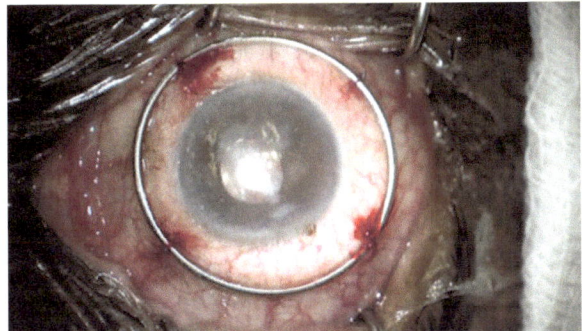

Fig. 26.4 Radial marker.
(Courtesy of Katena
instruments)

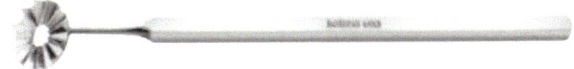

Marking the Eye for Suture Placement and Trephine Centration

Because the donor cornea is secured to the patient's cornea by sutures, proper placement of sutures is critical to both achieve good wound closure and to decrease irregular wound alignment. For example, if the donor cornea is not aligned properly with the patient's cornea, the wound may leak. If some sutures are askew or excessively tight, the resulting cornea shape will be irregular, causing distorted vision. Suturing the donor cornea to the patient's cornea involves placement of interrupted sutures, which are single sutures placed radially. This may be done with 16 interrupted sutures or with fewer interrupted sutures combined with a continuous running suture. Meticulous placement of interrupted sutures is critical for good wound closure and visual outcome.

To help guide suturing, most surgeons pre-place marks for suture placement. Typically, a gentian violet marking pen is used to mark the geometric center of the cornea. Then a special marker, which is a spoke-like instrument that has either 12 or 16 dull blades, is painted with gentian violet marking pen and gently applied onto the cornea. This would leave 12 or 16 radial marks to guide suture placement (Figs. 26.4 and 26.5).

Determining Transplant Size

In penetrating keratoplasty, the diseased portion of the patient's cornea is removed with a special blade. The instrument used to incise the patient's cornea is termed a trephine, which is a cylinder with a sharp blade at one end. A trephine will fashion a circular cut and it comes in varying diameters. Most donor trephines have a suction

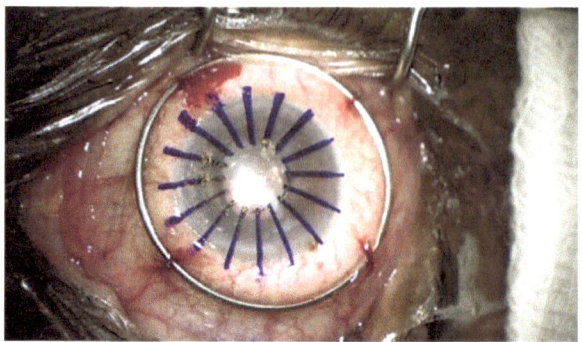

Fig. 26.5 Cornea with marks placed to guide sutures. (Our stock image)

apparatus that holds the donor tissue in place and a round trephine blade with metal posts which guide the trephine downwards to fashion the donor button (Fig. 26.6a). Host tissue trephines (Fig. 26.6b) are attached to a suction apparatus that allows it to be firmly secured to the eye by vacuum and have plastics spokes that can be easily turned to advance the blade. Trephines may also be freehand, in which the surgeon turns the trephine by hand while applying it onto the patient's cornea to achieve the incision (Fig. 26.7). The diameter of the trephination is dependent on the diameter of the cornea and the extent of the corneal pathology.

Your surgeon will use calipers to measure the size of the trephination to be performed (Fig. 26.8). This is often determined based on the minimal diameter required to remove all of the pathology as well as to achieve balance between small transplant diameter (which induces more astigmatism or irregular shape of the cornea) and large transplant diameter (which increases risk of glaucoma and rejection of the transplant). After deciding the size of the trephination for the patient, your surgeon will then decide the size of the trephination for the donor cornea. Often, the donor cornea will require a trephine that is 0.25 mm larger than the patient cornea. This slight oversize ensures good wound closure with sutures. In some cases, such as in pediatric keratoplasty, the oversize may be even larger. In other cases, such as for keratoconus patients, the donor cornea may be the same size as the patient's cornea to reduce postoperative myopia (nearsightedness).

Your surgeon may have already preselected the trephine type and size and brought the appropriate trephines into the room. In some instances, however, the decision is made on the table after measuring the patient's cornea with calipers. Here, the surgeon will indicate to the circulator which trephine is required. Your surgeon may say "Moria trephine 8.5 mm and Barron suction 8.25 mm " which indicates that for the donor cornea, he/she will use an 8.5 mm Moria trephine and for the patient's cornea, an 8.25 mm Barron suction trephine. By convention, the surgeon will ask for the larger donor trephine first and the smaller host cornea trephine second. Pay close attention to the type and size of trephines required as obtaining the wrong trephine may cause an unnecessary delay as the circulator would need to search again for the correct ones. In the worst-case scenario, the surgeon may use the wrong trephine and be faced with the unpleasant task of suturing a donor cornea that is too small for the patient.

Fig. 26.6 (**a**) Barron donor corneal punch. (**b**) Barron vacuum trephine. (Courtesy of Katena instruments)

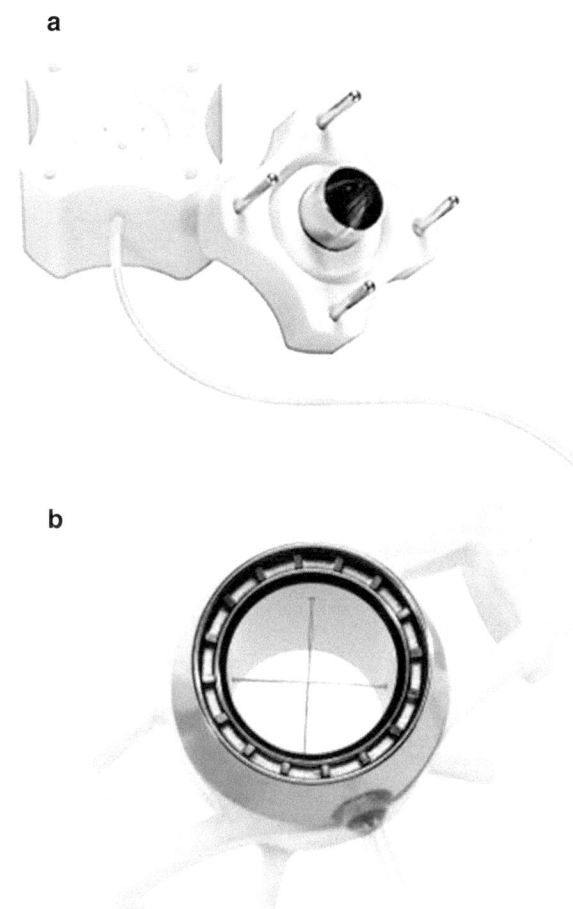

a

b

Once the circulator becomes familiar with the surgeon's preference of types of trephine, the surgeon may simply say "8.5 and 8.25." It is important to note that the larger size always refers to the trephine for the donor tissue. When in doubt, however, always confirm with the surgeon. Many surgical OR suites will keep a cart on

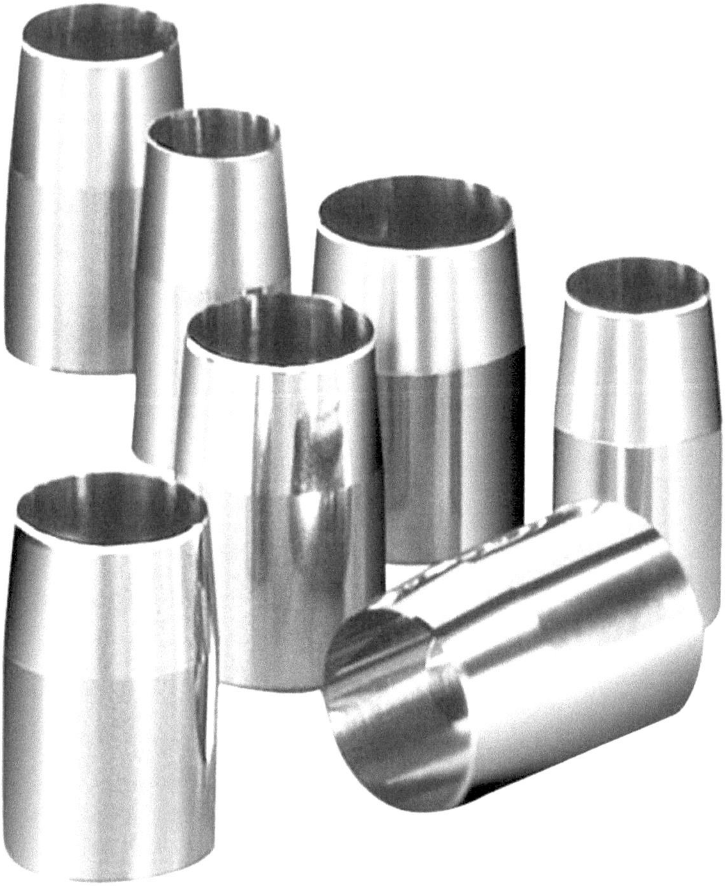

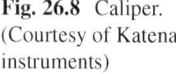

Fig. 26.7 Katena handheld trephines. (Courtesy of Katena instruments)

Fig. 26.8 Caliper.
(Courtesy of Katena
instruments)

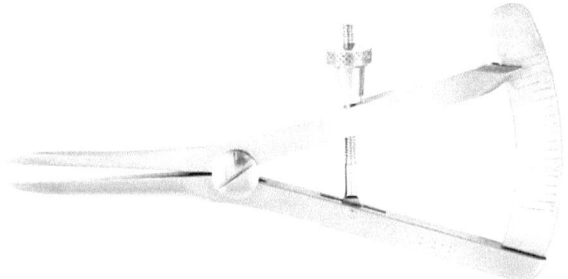

wheels that contains multiple sizes of trephines so the circulating nurse doesn't have to exit the room when the surgeon is measuring a patients eye when on the surgical table.

Preparing the Donor Cornea

Your surgeon will prepare the donor cornea prior to cutting the patient's cornea. This is to ensure that if the donor cornea trephination was faulty and the donor cornea cannot be used, there is still an option of not trephinating the host cornea and cancelling the surgery for that day.

A sterile side table would have been set up for donor cornea preparation. A separate table is typically set aside as the setup for cutting the donor cornea is bulky and best separated from the rest of the surgical instruments. This side table is covered with a sterile drape and set up with the instrumentation for the particular trephine. The circulating nurse will ensure that an overhead spotlight is placed over the table as the surgeon will need to see fine details during the preparation. The typical instruments on the side table include a .12 toothed forcep to grasp the tissue, a 5 cc syringe to aspirate extra cornea storage solution, and Weck cell sponges.

Your surgeon will call for the donor cornea tissue. The circulator will verbally confirm that the tissue is being opened and the specification, typically by announcing the unique eye bank ID (identification number on the container (Fig. 26.9). The circulator will then break the seal on the container, carefully unscrew the top, and tilt

Fig. 26.9 PK tissue in Krolman container. (Our Image)

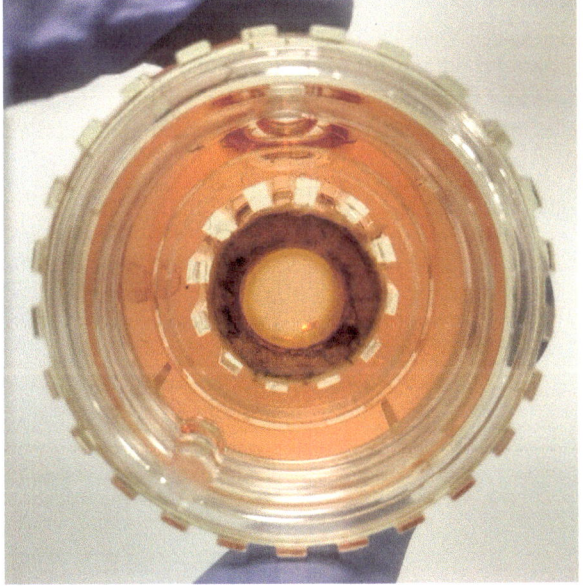

the container toward the surgeon while steadying it with both hands above the side table. The surgeon will then grasp the cornea by the rim with a toothed forceps and place it on the trephine. The surgeon will also withdraw a small amount of cornea storage solution from the container using a 3 cc syringe to lubricate the donor cornea.

The donor cornea is then cut or trephinated using the suction trephine. The cornea is placed endothelial side up, the vacuum is applied to avoid tissue slippage, and then the trephine either pressed or rotated down to achieve the circular cut. The trephinated cornea is then coated with cornea storage media to prevent desiccation. The residual rim of the donor cornea is typically sent for microbiology cultures. The surgeon or the scrub technician will place the rim into a thioglycolate broth tube, and the donor rim will be sent off to the microbiology laboratory.

Trephinating the Patient Cornea

Your surgeon will then trephinate the patient's cornea. A suction trephine is typically employed. The trephine is applied with even pressure to the eye. The surgeon will indicate when suction is to be applied. At this point, the assistant, which could be the scrub technician, depresses on the plunger of the attached 5 cc syringe and then quickly releases to build vacuum. Commonly, the plunger will stop between the 4 and 5 cc mark to indicate proper suction. Your surgeon confirms suction is present, that is, the trephine is now securely attached to the eye without slippage. The surgeon then performs the trephination until the eye is entered which is indicated with an egress of aqueous fluid.

Your surgeon will request viscoelastic to place below the cornea. This serves to protect the iris and lens from inadvertent injury during cutting of the cornea. The circular cornea button will then be removed using either corneal scissors (a pair, termed right and left corneal scissors to indicate whether they cut counterclockwise or clockwise) or a diamond trifacet blade (Fig. 26.10). To steady the cornea during the cut, your surgeon may grasp the cornea with 0.12 forceps or Girard or Colibri

Fig. 26.10 (**a**) Diamond trifacet blade. (**b**) Magnify tip. (Katena)

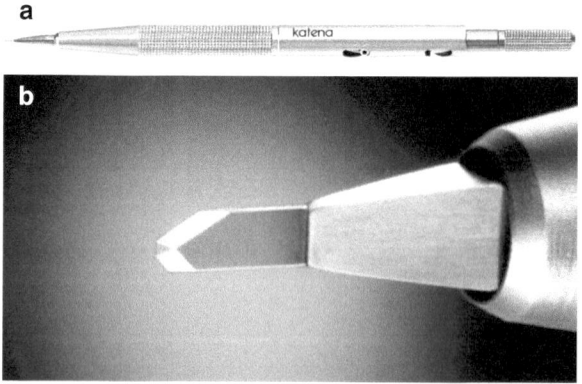

forceps (modified 0.12 forceps with the end angled to allow for easy grasp of cornea). The freed cornea button is then handed off to the scrub's technician. The cornea button is then sent off to pathology for histologic examination. In cases of infection, the surgeon will commonly bisect the host cornea and send half the cornea to microbiology and the other half to pathology.

Suturing the Cornea

Once the patient's cornea is removed, time is of the essence. "Open sky," a term used to refer to an eye that is open and unprotected by cornea tissue, puts the patient at risk of a suprachoroidal or expulsive hemorrhage, an often devastating complication. Your surgeon will therefore work expeditiously to "close" the eye by suturing the donor cornea onto the patient efficiently. The donor cornea, now resting on the trephine block, is handed carefully to the surgeon. The surgeon then requests a tissue spatula or spoon (Fig. 26.11), which is used to scoop up the cornea. The donor cornea is then placed, endothelial side down, on the patient's eye.

Typically, 10-0 nylon sutures are used to suture a corneal transplant (Fig. 26.12). These sutures will be evenly placed in a radial fashion, much like the hours of a clock. If only single sutures (also termed interrupted sutures) are used, typically 16 sutures will be placed. Alternatively, one or more continuous 10-0 nylon sutures may be placed in a purse string fashion, or interrupted sutures may be combined with a running suture. Most corneal surgeons prefer a spatulated needle. This is a needle with a flattened, reverse cutting point, with the third cutting edge on the bottom removed. The flattened configuration easily splits the corneal lamellae and is minimally traumatic. The most common needles are the Alcon CU-5 and the Ethicon 160-0 needle configurations.

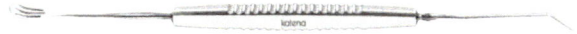

Fig. 26.11 Issue spatula. (Courtesy of Katena instruments)

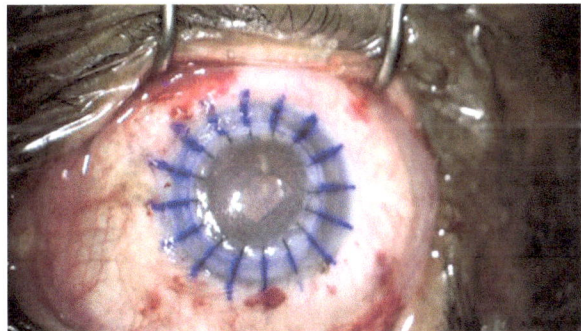

Fig. 26.12 PK with 16 interrupted sutures. (Our stock image)

Fig. 26.13 Loading needle
(**a**) forehand (**b**) backhand.
(Scrubs Bible Ver 1)

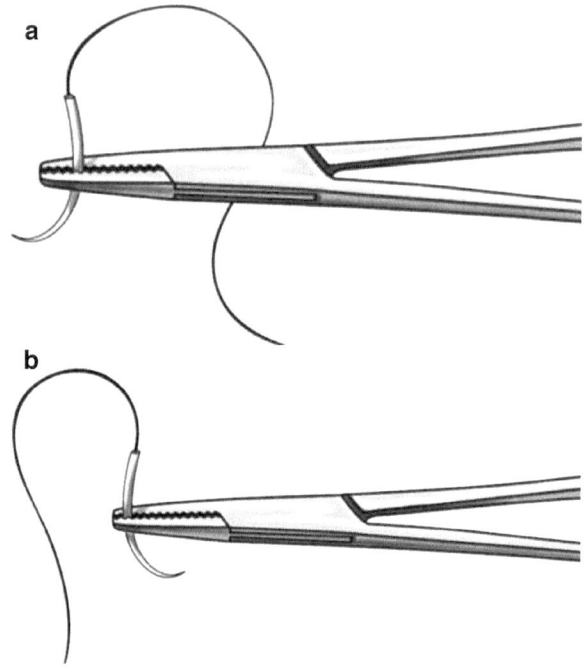

Some of the sutures will require the needle to be loaded forehand, and others will require the needle to be loaded backhand (Fig. 26.13). Your surgeon may alternate loading the needle him/herself. Alternatively, your surgeon may prefer that you load it. If you are required to load the needle each time, have a second needle driver that you can load while the first is being use. In between the passage and tying of each suture, you would need to pass the Vannas scissors to the surgeon to cut the suture. Depending on the surgeon's speed, the suturing process may require rapid alternation between loading needles, passing scissors, or even tying forceps. Lapses of attention during this process should be avoided.

Figure 26.14, SuperScrub master of passing needle.

Concluding the Case

Once the suturing is complete, your surgeon and you may take a breath as there is no further risk of the "open sky" situation. After the suturing is completed, your surgeon will request tying forceps to bury the knots. Burying the knots refers to rotating the

Fig. 26.14 SuperScrub is a master at passing the needle holder efficiently to a waiting surgeon

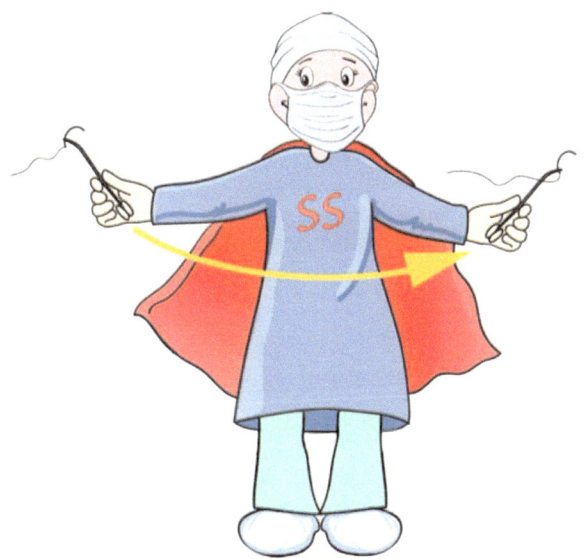

suture so that the knot is inside the cornea tissue as opposed to on the surface. Unburied sutures cause irritation, discomfort, and light sensitivity and may be a nidus for infection. Tying forceps are always non-toothed and allow for manipulating the sutures without breaking them. At the end of the procedure, the surgeon will frequently inject balanced salt solution on a cannula to deepen the anterior chamber and restore the normal integrity of the globe. The Flieringa ring, if used, will also be removed.

Your surgeon will check the integrity of the wound, either by depressing circumferentially with a ophthalmic sponge or by applying a fluorescein strip to the wound to check for a leak. Occasionally, an additional suture(s) will need to be replaced either due to breakage or nonuniform tension. If your surgeon is satisfied with the suturing, the case is then concluded typically with subconjunctival injection or topical irrigation of antibiotics and steroids.

At the conclusion of the case, be sure that all needles opened during the surgery are accounted for. If a needle is lost during the procedure, gently inform your surgeon so that he/she can search the surgical field for the missing needle. At times, the

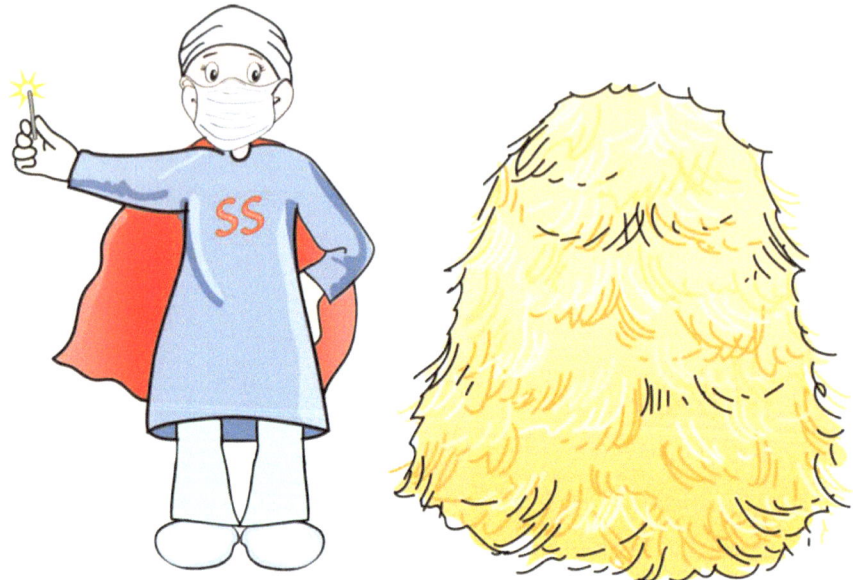

Fig. 26.15 SuperScrub doesn't get caught searching for unaccounted for needles in a haystack

needle may be caught on the speculum or fallen onto the drape or into the side pocket used to collect fluids. Leaving a needle around or in the patient's eye at the conclusion of surgery is not permissible. The surgical tray for penetrating keratoplasty cases is found in Chap. 33.

Figure 26.15 shows SuperScrub finding a needle in a haystack.

Chapter 27
Corneal Transplantation: Keratoprosthesis

A keratoprosthesis surgery is corneal transplantation using an artificial cornea. This is in contrast to a traditional penetrating keratoplasty (described previously) that utilizes the cornea from a deceased donor. A keratoprosthesis (also abbreviated as Kpro) is used in situations where using a donor cornea is unlikely to succeed. To be successful, transplanted donor corneas would need to clear following the keratoplasty. In cases where the cornea does not clear or initially clears but becomes cloudy later on, the transplant is said to have failed.

Certain patient characteristics predispose penetrating keratoplasty performed using donor cornea at high risk for failing. For instance, if the patient has had multiple prior corneal transplants, severe dry eye, scar formation (also called synechiae formation) in the eye, or significant vessel ingrowth on the cornea, he/she is at risk of failure following a traditional penetrating keratoplasty. Your surgeon may decide, based on the patient's history and clinical exam that a traditional keratoplasty using a donor cornea is unlikely to lead to long-term success. An alternative would be performing a keratoplasty using an artificial cornea, or keratoprosthesis.

There are various types and materials of keratoprosthesis and techniques of implantation. In generally, keratoprosthesis is made of a clear plastic optic that is attached to human donor tissue. Because the keratoprosthesis has a central optic area comprised of inert plastic, there is no risk of central opacification from corneal swelling or scarring. You may ask, why then do surgeons not use keratoprosthesis as the primary procedure for corneal transplantation? Although the central optic of a keratoprosthesis has no risk of opacification, the KPro apparatus is associated with a higher postoperative complication rate. These postoperative complications include but are not limited to retroprosthetic membrane formation, glaucoma, tissue melting, and postoperative infection, among others. Therefore, the criteria for keratoprosthesis surgery are very selective.

Although several keratoprosthesis devices have been developed, the mostly common used devices is the Boston keratoprosthesis so named because it was developed in Boston. The Boston keratoprosthesis (BKpro) is made of medical grade polymethylmethacrylate (PMMA) and consists of a front plate with a stem, a back plate,

© Springer Nature Switzerland AG 2020   163
R. S. Koplin et al., *The Scrub's Bible*,
https://doi.org/10.1007/978-3-030-44345-0_27

and a locking ring. There are two types of Boston keratoprosthesis. Type 1 kerato-prosthesis is implanted much like a traditional keratoplasty. The Type 2 keratopros-thesis has a longer stem that protrudes through the eyelid and is used in patients with severe dry eyes. A Type 1 keratoprosthesis is much more commonly used and will be discussed herein.

Recently, there have been upgrades in the Type 1 keratoprosthesis model back plates. A larger diameter titanium back plate to clamp the donor-host junction has been introduced to decrease the rate of retroprosthetic membrane formation (RPM) compared to standard PMMA back plates. Secondly, there are now two types of back plate attachments. A newer titanium threadless "click-on" type that clicks onto the optic of the front plate and does not require a locking ring and the traditional "snap-on" type made from either PMMA or titanium that is further secured with a titanium locking ring. The older "snap-on" type has back plate options of 7.0 mm or 8.5 mm in diameter.

The Operation

The basic principle of keratoprosthesis surgery is full-thickness removal of patient's cornea and replacement with a keratoprosthesis (Fig. 27.1).

The initial steps of keratoprosthesis surgery are identical to penetrating kerato-plasty. Your surgeon may elect to stabilize the eye with Fleiringa ring and place marks for suture placement. Next, your surgeon will determine the size of trephina-tion for the patient and for the donor cornea. Please refer to Chap. 26 Penetrating Keratoplasty for a description of these steps: stabilizing the eye, marking the eye for suture placement, and determining transplant size.

Preparing the Donor Cornea and Assembling the Keratoprosthesis

Although an artificial cornea is used in keratoprosthesis surgery, a donor cornea is still required. This donor cornea will be sandwiched in between the front optic and the back plate of the keratoprosthesis. The donor cornea allows for suturing to the patient's cornea (imagine trying to suture plastic to the eye without it!) and a tighter wound seal.

Your surgeon will prepare the donor cornea on a sterile side table with the appro-priate trephine set up. Your surgeon will call for the donor cornea tissue. The circu-lator will verbally confirm that the tissue is being opened and the specification (typically by announcing the unique eye bank ID number on the container). The circulator will then break the seal on the container, carefully unscrew the top, and tilt the container toward the surgeon while steadying it with both hands above the

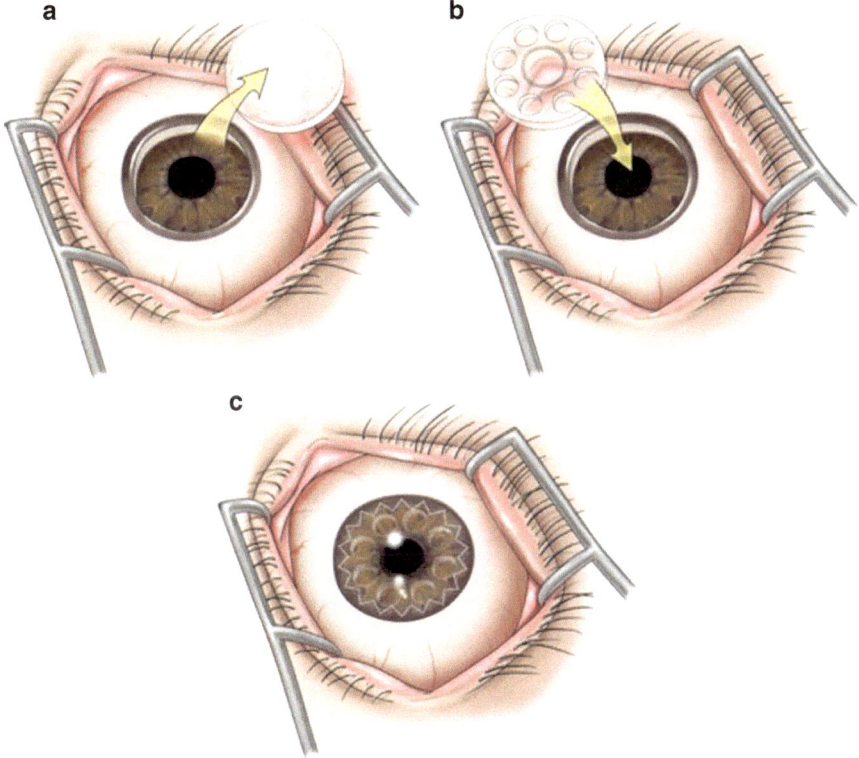

Fig. 27.1 (**a–c**) Keratoprosthesis schematic. (**a**) Removal of diseased cornea. (**b**) Replacement with keratoprosthesis. (**c**) Keratoprosthesis secured with sutures

side table. The surgeon will then grasp the tissue with toothed forceps and place it on the trephine. The surgeon will also withdraw a small amount of cornea storage solution from the container using a 3 cc syringe to wet the cornea. The donor cornea is then trephinated using the trephine. This typically involves a suction trephine. The tissue is placed endothelial side up, the vacuum is applied to avoid tissue slippage, and then the trephine either pressed or rotated down to achieve the circular cut.

As you may have noticed, the preparation of the donor cornea is thus far identical to that in penetrating keratoplasty. In keratoprosthesis surgery, there are additional steps. The donor cornea needs to be held in place between the front plate optic and the back plate of the keratoprosthesis. This is performed by creating a central 3 mm hole in the donor cornea button using a 3 mm donor punch provided in the keratoprosthesis assembly package. To do so, your surgeon will use a 3 mm dermatological punch (contained in the keratoprosthesis package) to fashion a full-thickness hole in the center of the cornea button. The cornea button now looks essentially like a donut (typically 8–9 mm wide with a central 3 mm hole).

Next, your surgeon will assemble the keratoprosthesis (Fig. 27.2). The keratoprosthesis package consists of a non-sterile outer envelope with a sterile inner

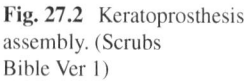

Fig. 27.2 Keratoprosthesis
assembly. (Scrubs
Bible Ver 1)

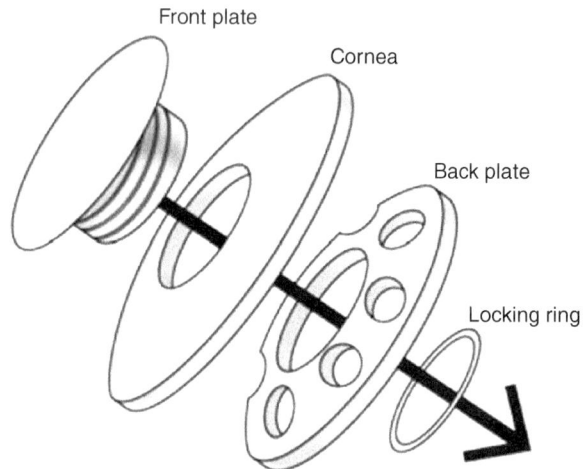

envelope containing the keratoprosthesis components. The circulator will open the
non-sterile envelope, exposing the inner envelope to the surgeon who can then grasp
it in a sterile fashion. Your surgeon will then assemble the keratoprosthesis in this
order: front plate optic, donor cornea, back plate, and titanium locking ring. He/she
will place the assembled keratoprosthesis unit in tissue storage solution to prevent
desiccation.

Remember that the residual rim of the donor cornea is typically sent for microbiology cultures. The surgeon or the scrub technician will place the rim into a thioglycolate broth held by the circulator and sent off to microbiology.

Trephinating the Patient's Cornea and Removing
Intraocular Lens

Following the assembly of the keratoprosthesis, your surgeon will then trephinate
the patient's cornea. Please refer to Chap. 26 Penetrating Keratoplasty for a description of this step. For patients who have an intraocular lens implant, your surgeon
may elect to remove the lens implant prior to securing the keratoprosthesis. The
optic (central clear portion of the keratoprosthesis) comes in different powers and
therefore can also replace the focusing power of an intraocular lens implant.

If your surgeon elects to remove an intraocular lens implant, he/she will grasp it
with a Kelman forceps and in some cases may amputate (or cut) the haptics of the
lens implant using scissors if the haptics are incarcerated into the anterior chamber
angle. The lens implant would then be sent off to pathology. Often, following
removal of an intraocular lens, your surgeon will perform an anterior vitrectomy to
remove any vitreous that may have been brought forward during intraocular lens
removal.

To prepare the vitrectomy system, you will simply set up the vitrectomy hand-piece, set the console for vitrectomy, set aspiration and cutting as determined by your surgeon, and run the infusion through the line, ridding the system of air bubbles. If the system is a split device – infusion handpiece and cutting handpiece separate – the tubes will likewise be split between the two instruments.

Suturing the Keratoprosthesis

A keratoprosthesis is sutured to the patient's eye much like a donor cornea in penetrating keratoplasty. Your surgeon will use 10-0 nylon sutures placed in a radial fashion. Almost always 16 interrupted sutures are employed. Be ready to load the needle alternating backhand and forehand as needed. Your surgeon will request tying forceps to bury the knots.

Concluding the Case

Once the suturing is complete, your surgeon will check the integrity of the wound, either by depressing circumferentially with Weck-cell sponges or by applying a fluorescein strip to the wound to check for wound leak. Occasionally, a suture would need to be replaced either due to breakage or nonuniform tension. If your surgeon is satisfied with the transplant, the case is then concluded typically with subconjunctival injection or topical irrigation of antibiotics and steroids. In addition, a contact lens will be placed over the keratoprosthesis to keep the ocular surface from desiccating. The surgical tray for keratoprosthesis cases is found in Chap. 34.

Figure 27.3 is a clinical image of keratoprosthesis.

Fig. 27.3 Keratoprosthesis picture. (Our image)

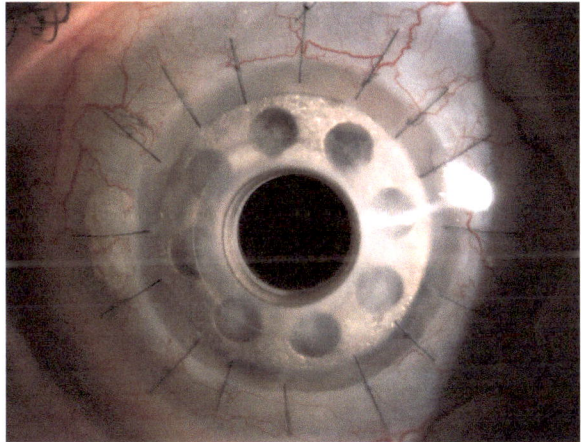

Chapter 28
Corneal Transplantation: Endothelial Keratoplasty/DSAEK

Background

The last two decades has heralded a revolutionary shift in the treatment of corneal endothelial disease. Previously, the only surgical treatment for corneal edema due to Fuchs' dystrophy or pseudophakic bullous keratopathy was a full-thickness penetrating keratoplasty. Although full-thickness corneal transplantation has been widely successful for many decades, it requires months of refractive adjustments before the eyes can achieve visual stability. This evolutionary change has seen the number of endothelial corneal transplants in the United States rise from just over 6000 in 2006 to nearly 31,000 in 2018. Endothelial keratoplasty (EK) enables the surgical treatment of corneal endothelial disease with less extensive surgery, faster visual recovery, less corneal irregularity induced by suturing, a lower risk of rejection, and improved globe stability as compared to traditional penetrating keratoplasty (PK). The EK procedure selectively replaces only the inner layers of the cornea, i.e., the endothelium. Because of these advantages, EK is the preferred operation over PK when only the endothelium of the patient's cornea is diseased. Each new iteration of endothelial keratoplasty has involved the increasingly selective transplantation of corneal endothelial cells.

The most commonly performed type of EK is Descemet stripping endothelial keratoplasty (DSEK), also referred to as Descemet stripping automated endothelial keratoplasty (DSAEK) (the automated refers to the donor tissue being prepared using a microkeratome as opposed to by hand). In DSAEK a small portion of donor stromal tissue (generally 120 microns or less) along with the Descemet's membrane and the endothelial cell layer are transplanted to the host cornea. Following the widespread adoption of DSAEK surgery, a new evolutionary technique coined DMEK (Descemet's membrane endothelial keratoplasty) transplantation was developed. In DMEK, the donor Descemet's membrane minus the 120 microns less of donor corneal stroma is stripped from a corneoscleral rim and injected into the host anterior segment that has been stripped of its own Descemet's membrane. The

© Springer Nature Switzerland AG 2020
R. S. Koplin et al., *The Scrub's Bible*,
https://doi.org/10.1007/978-3-030-44345-0_28

membrane is unfurled within the anterior chamber using pneumatic and fluid manipulations as in DSAEK. The DMEK tissue is then apposed to the recipient posterior stroma using either air of sulfur hexafluoride (SF6) gas for tamponade to host stroma. A 3–3.25 mm clear corneal incision is employed.

DSAEK

The Operation

The basic principle of DSAEK is partial thickness removal of patient's cornea and replacement with partial thickness donor cornea (Fig. 28.1).

Donor Tissue Preparation

In DSAEK, donor tissue preparation involves two steps: lamellar dissection to separate the inner layers of the cornea (deep stroma and endothelium) from the outer layers (epithelium and superficial stroma) and trephination to create a circular shape. The first step, lamellar dissection, is now typically performed using a microkeratome, an instrument that removes a thin layer of tissue from the cornea. In the last decade, this step is primarily performed by the eye bank. Nearly all DSAEK tissue in the United States arrives "precut" from the Eyebank and this step is rarely ever performed by your surgeon.

In most cases the donor tissue has been premarked by the eye bank with three lines to allow alignment of the lamellar cap and the donor tissue. This allows the

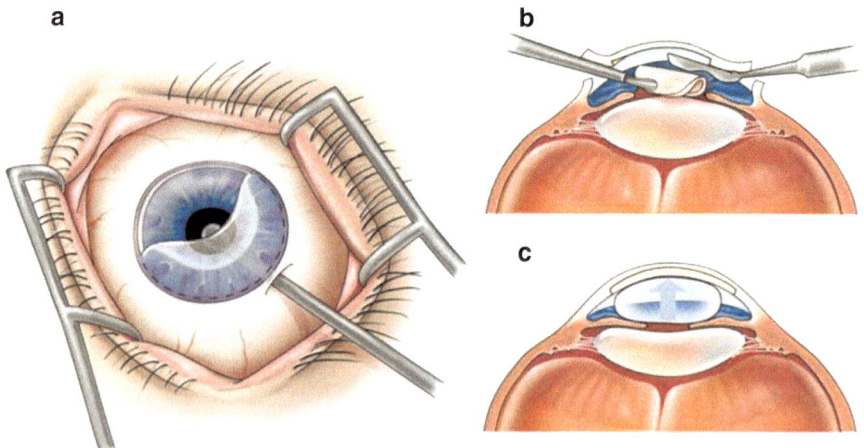

Fig. 28.1 (**a–c**) DSAEK schematic (**a**) removal of Descemet's membrane. (**b**) Insertion of donor lenticule. (**c**) Attachment of donor lenticule to recipient using air bubble

Fig. 28.2 Premarked
DSAEK in Krolman
viewing chamber.
(Our image)

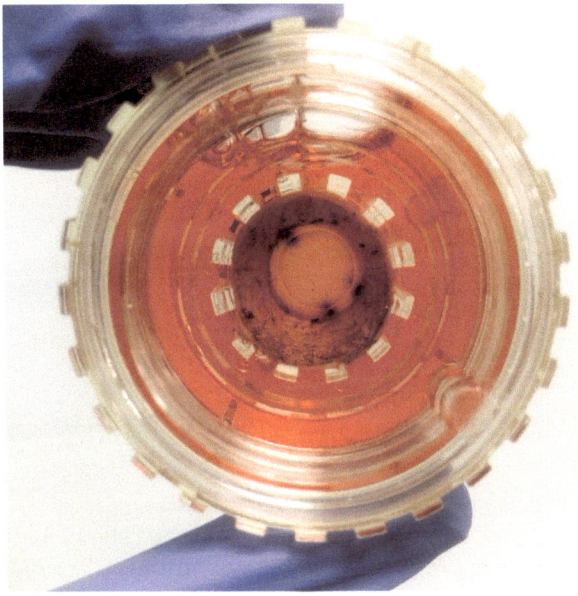

surgery to differentiate the lamellar cap from the donor lenticule (Fig. 28.2). The precut tissue (cap and lenticule) lamellar dissection of the donor cornea (to leave only the posterior stroma and endothelium), the cornea is then trephinated to the desired size. This typically involves a suction trephine. The tissue is placed endothelial side up, the vacuum is applied to avoid tissue slippage, and then the trephine either pressed or rotated down to achieve the circular cut. The cornea button is then covered with tissue storage solution to prevent desiccation (drying).

Removing the patient's Descemet's Membrane

After donor tissue preparation, your surgeon will turn his/her attention to the patient. The first step of the surgery will involve removal of the Descemet's membrane from the patient's cornea. Although the exact technique may vary according to surgeon preference, generally, this step involves the creation of one or more paracenteses using a 15 degree blade or a diamond paracentesis blade. Some surgeon may insert an anterior chamber maintainer to supply a controllable volume of balanced salt solution into the eye to prevent collapse of the anterior chamber. Others may inject viscoelastic or air instead to maintain the anterior chamber.

Your surgeon will request a reverse Sinskey hook, an instrument with a dull or blunted hook at one end. With the reverse Sinskey hook (Fig. 28.3), your surgeon will score the Descemet's membrane in a circular fashion. Some surgeons often pre-place a circular mark on the patient's cornea using an optic zone marker with gentian violet to provide a guide for scoring (Fig. 28.4). Once the scoring of the

Fig. 28.3 Endoscorer.
(Moria)

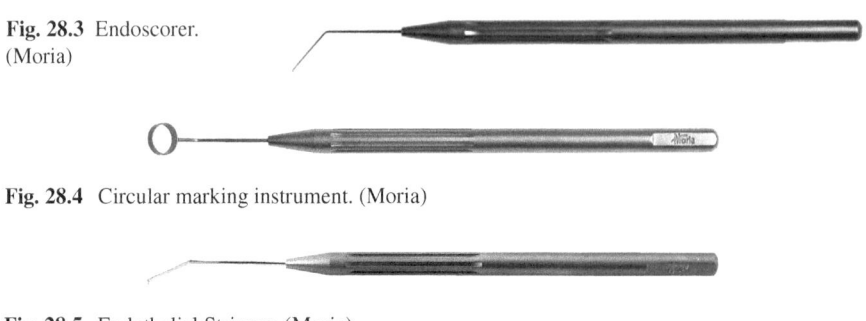

Fig. 28.4 Circular marking instrument. (Moria)

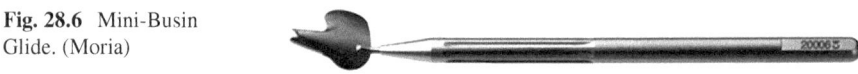

Fig. 28.5 Endothelial Stripper. (Moria)

Fig. 28.6 Mini-Busin
Glide. (Moria)

endothelium is complete, your surgeon will request a keratome to create a corneal incision. This incision, typically 4–5 mm, allows for the removal of the Descemet's membrane from the eye and the subsequent insertion of the donor graft. Rarely, some surgeons may elect to create a scleral tunnel incision. This would involve exposing the sclera by creating incisions in the conjunctiva using Westcott scissors, cauterizing the scleral bed to tamponade any bleeding, and then using a blade such as crescent blade to create the scleral tunnel. Your surgeon will use an endothelial stripper or rake (Fig. 28.5), an instrument with a rake at the end, to remove the Descemet's membrane that is then sent off to pathology in a container with formalin. If viscoelastic is used to maintain the anterior chamber during Descemet's membrane removal, then an irrigation handpiece connected to a phacoemulsification machine will be needed to remove all the viscoelastic placed prior to stripping.

Inserting the Donor Cornea

Once the patient's Descemet's membrane has been removed, your surgeon is now ready to insert the donor cornea. There are several ways to insert the donor cornea: folding (in which the cornea is folded in a taco shape with DSAEK lamellar inserting forceps and deposited into the anterior chamber) or with a variety of commercially available inserters. These inserters may be single use or reusable. Generally, these inserters have a small platform in the shape of a spoon that holds the cornea, and then the cornea edges are rolled up so that the cornea can be inserted into the anterior chamber via a small incision. Once in the anterior chamber, the donor cornea may still be in a furled position or spontaneously unfurl. If not, your surgeon will inject balanced salt solution via a 27 gauge cannula through a paracentesis tract to unfurl the donor cornea.

Figure 28.6 shows a mini-Busin endothelial glide.

Fig. 28.7 Air bubble. (Our
stock image)

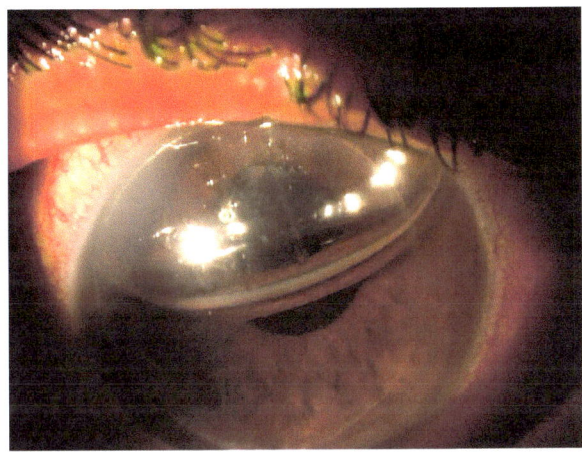

Attaching the Donor Cornea

The donor cornea will be free-floating in the anterior chamber. Attachment of the donor cornea to the patient's cornea is critical for the success of the surgery. Your surgeon will first close the main incision followed by any leaking paracenteses wounds with 10-0 nylon sutures to ensure an air tight seal. Your surgeon will then ask for a 27 gauge cannula and inject the air slowly but deliberately through the paracentesis tract. The air bubble floats to the top and will force the donor cornea against the patient's cornea, allowing for attachment (Fig. 28.7). Some surgeons request a drop of a long-acting dilating agent such as cyclopentolate, homatropine, or atropine to be placed in the eye. This serves to dilate the pupil so that air does not migrate and becomes trapped behind the iris, causing a condition called pupillary block that can lead to high eye pressure and pain. Other surgeons prefer a miotic agent to constrict the pupil, which also prevents migration of the air behind the iris.

Concluding the Case

After a short period of time to allow the donor cornea to attach, your surgeon may remove some air to prevent pupillary block. He/she will do so with a 27 gauge cannula or 30 gauge needle. At the conclusion of the surgery, a mixture of antibiotics and steroids is typically either irrigated onto the eye or injected in the subconjunctival space. Following the surgery, the patient is instructed to remain flat, often until the next day (except for necessary short breaks). This includes the time while in the recovery area before discharge. Often, a sign indicating that the patient had a DSAEK procedure and needs to remain flat until discharge is placed on the surgical stretcher.

Figure 28.8 shows SuperScrub holding a sign to lay flat.

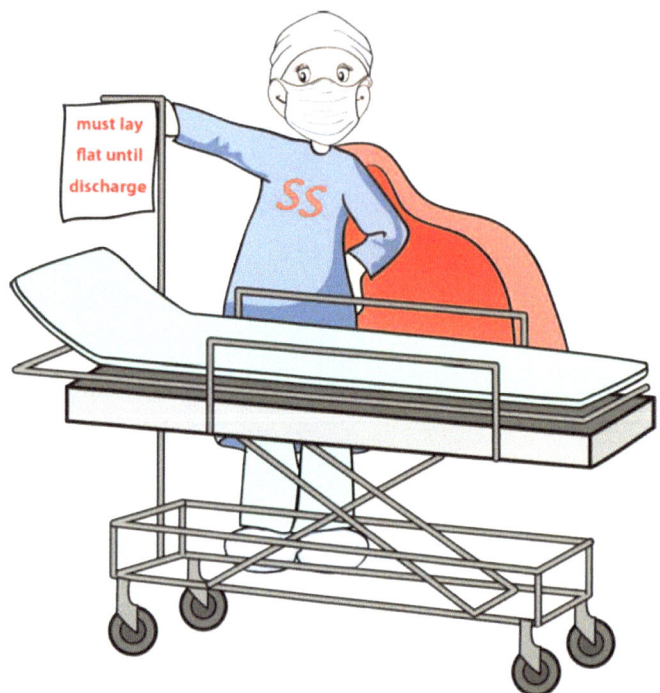

Fig. 28.8 SuperScrub remind patients to lay flat following DSAEK operation

Chapter 29
Corneal Transplantation: Endothelial Keratoplasty/DMEK

Background

Descemet stripping automated endothelial keratoplasty (DSAEK) in less than a decade has virtually eliminated the use of full-thickness keratoplasty to treat diseases of the endothelial layer. Corneal surgeons have embraced DSAEK as a quick, highly successful surgery to replace diseased endothelial cells. However, while the residual stroma on the endothelial cells gives the tissue some rigidity that makes it easier to implant, it may result in a refractive shift, cause a small loss of best corrected visual acuity, and still may result in a higher rate of graft rejection then desired. As such, DMEK was developed as an alternative approach to endothelial keratoplasty to address these specific issues. Studies have found that postoperative visual acuity is 1–2 lines better on average, that the refractive shift is almost eliminated, and that the risk of rejection is lower than DSAEK. However, the procedure may be technically challenging due to the "no touch" method, and the rates of postoperative detachment of the donor tissue are sometimes higher.

The initial events of the procedure are similar to DSAEK. The first step of the surgery will involve removal of the Descemet's membrane from the patient's cornea. Although the exact technique may vary according to surgeon preference, generally, this step involves creating of one or more paracentesis using a 15 degree blade or a diamond paracentesis blade. Many surgeons may insert an anterior chamber maintainer to supply a controlled volume of balanced salt solution into the eye to prevent collapse of the anterior chamber.

Your surgeon will request a reverse Sinskey hook, an instrument with a dull or blunted hook at one end. With the reverse Sinskey hook, your surgeon will score the Descemet's membrane in a circular fashion. Some surgeons may have pre-placed a circular mark on the patient's cornea using an optic zone marker with gentian violet to provide a guide for scoring. Unlike DSAEK, a peripheral iridotomy is created inferiorly in DMEK as the gas tends to sit superiorly when the patient is upright. Your surgeon will use two Sinskey hooks placed through inferior a superior

© Springer Nature Switzerland AG 2020
R. S. Koplin et al., *The Scrub's Bible*,
https://doi.org/10.1007/978-3-030-44345-0_29

paracenteses in a push-pull technique, to create a hole in the peripheral inferior iris. Some surgeons will perform a peripheral iridectomy prior to surgery in the office with a laser. The iridotomy prevents pupillary block from occurring postoperatively which is more likely in DMEK because of the use of sulfur hexafluoride gas (SF6) to tamponade the tissue as apposed to air that is most frequently used in DSAEK. Once the scoring of the endothelium and the iridotomy are complete, the BSS irrigation can be removed, and your surgeon will suture that paracentesis site. The surgeon will then request a keratome to create a 3.00–3.25 mm corneal incision for insertion of the tissue and removal of the scored Descemet's membrane tissue. The procedure differs from the DSAEK in a few ways.

1. Tissue preparation: Most eye banks are precutting donor DMEK tissue and pre-loading the DMEK tissue into a glass injector; however this is not yet universal. The eye bank will peel the endothelial cells and Descemet's membrane from the underlying stromal bed. The scroll is then immersed in a well of trypan blue and is stained for 4 minutes. An "F" or "S" mark is placed with a gentian violet marker to aid in orientation of the tissue. The prestripped, prestained, prestamped tissue is drawn into a Straiko Modified Jones glass tube (Gunther Weiss Scientific Glassblowing Co, Portland, Oregon) (Fig. 29.1) and placed in Optisol-GS solution inside a Krolman viewing chamber (Fig. 29.2).
2. In the operating room on a separate table, the DMEK tissue in the Straiko Modified Jones glass tube is removed from the Krolman view chamber. A 14 French precut catheter tubing (1.5 cm) with a male and female adapter (Fig. 29.3) is attached to a 5 cc syringe filled with BSS solution.
3. The syringe/catheter setup is then attached to the Straiko modified glass tubing.
4. The whole assembly is then placed into a petri dish filled with BSS, and a small amount of Optisol-GS™ is pressed out of the Modified Jones tube into the BSS well, and an equal amount of BSS is drawn into the tip. This is done to remove some of the Optisol-GS™ from the tissue so it is not injected into the eye.

Fig. 29.1 DMEK-tissue loaded in modified Straiko Jones tube. (Our image)

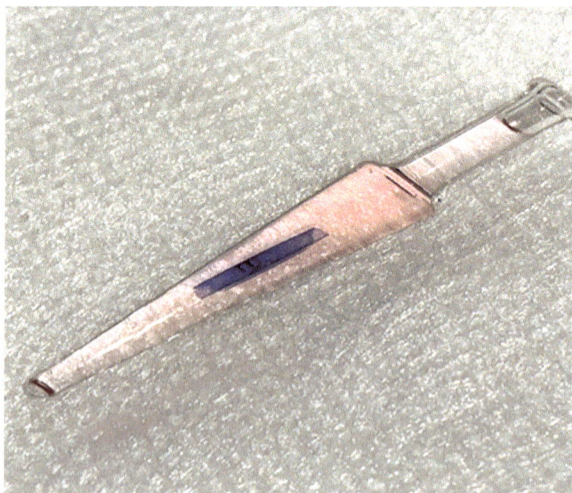

Fig. 29.2 DMEK in
Straiko Jones tube in
Krolman viewing chamber.
(Our image)

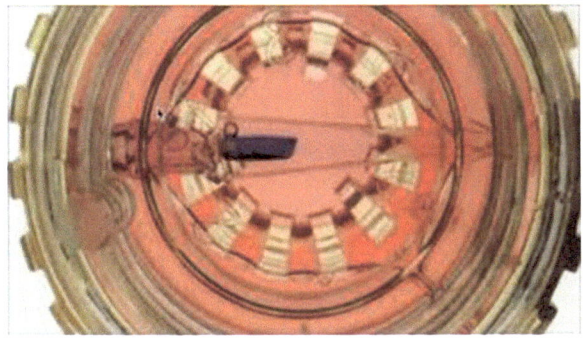

Fig. 29.3 Precut catheter
tubing with male/female
adaptor. (Our image)

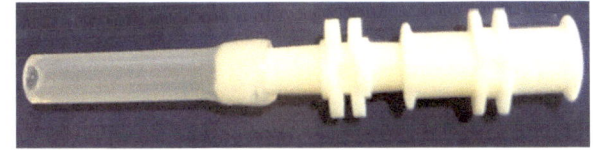

5. The modified Straiko Jones tube is placed through the wound bevel down, and
   the tissue is carefully injected through a 3.00–3.25 mm corneal incision taking
   care to keep the pressure in the anterior chamber low, so that the scroll does not
   eject through the corneal wounds. This is accomplished by having the surgical
   assistant press on a paracentesis to bleed aqueous out of the paracentesis to lower
   the IOP, while the DMEK graft is being inserted.
6. The scroll is unfurled after closing the wound with a 10-0 nylon suture. This
   process is done using a "tapping" technique, affectionately termed the "DMEK
   dance," whereby the tapping on the surface of the cornea causes flow of aqueous
   in a manner that encourages the graft to unfurl.
7. When the graft is correctly oriented (an "F" or "S" stamp is visible on the graft)
   and centered, 20% sulfur hexafluoride (SF6) gas is then injected under the graft
   to achieve an 80% fill.
8. To prepare the gas: Fill 10 cc syringe with air. Release 2 cc. Draw in 2 cc of 20%
   sulfur hexafluoride gas (SF6).

Chapter 30
Pterygium Surgery

A *pterygium* (Fig. 30.1) is a wing-shaped growth from the conjunctiva that invades onto the cornea. The term comes from the Greek word *ptergion* meaning "wing." It often appears as a yellowish or white elevated growth. A pterygium is a benign, i.e., noncancerous, growth. It is more common in dry, windy environments. It may also be related to ultraviolet light exposure. Several studies have shown a higher rate of pterygia in countries nearer the equator. A pterygium can be of no consequence, or it can cause irritation or interfere with vision if it invades far enough onto the cornea.

A patient may elect to have a pterygium removed due to cosmesis, irritation, or vision distortion. Pterygium surgery typically involves MAC sedation with regional anesthesia delivered in the form of retrobulbar anesthesia. Please refer to the anesthesia section for further details.

Fig. 30.1 Pterygium. (Our stock image)

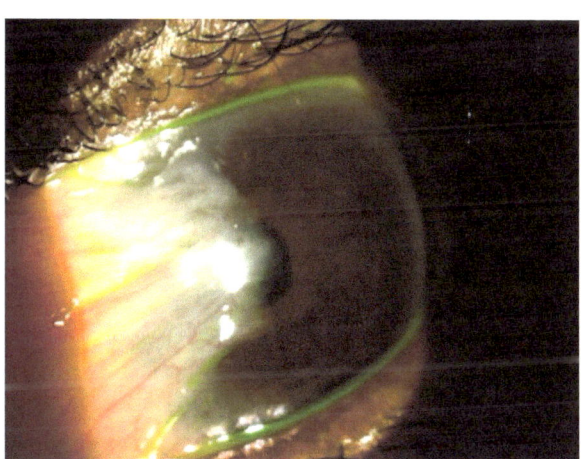

© Springer Nature Switzerland AG 2020
R. S. Koplin et al., *The Scrub's Bible*,
https://doi.org/10.1007/978-3-030-44345-0_30

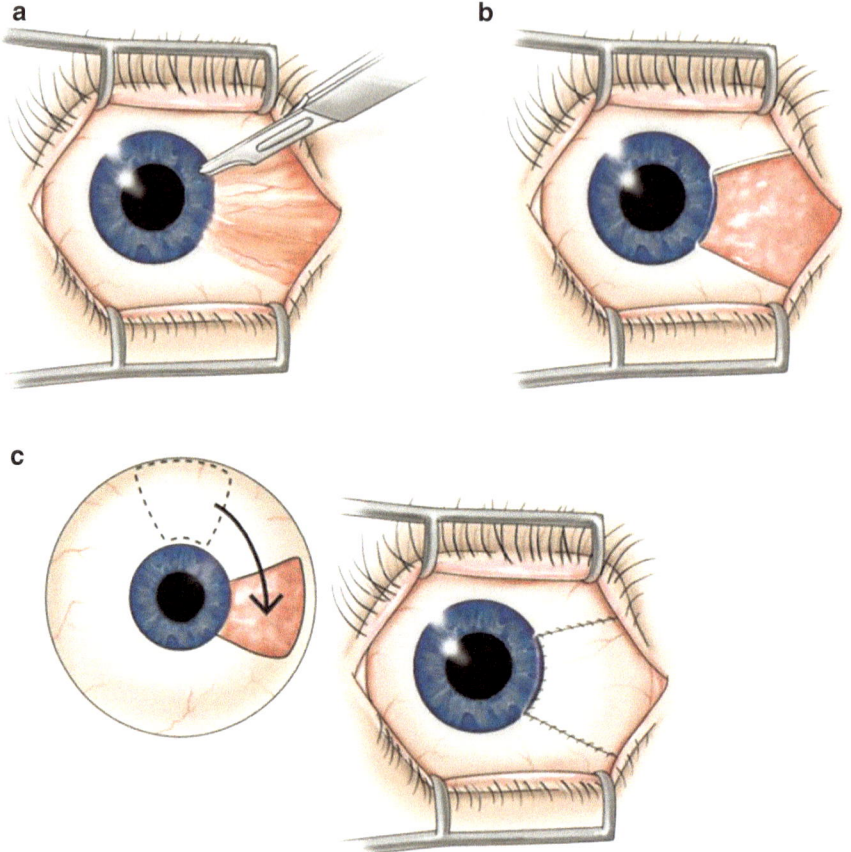

Fig. 30.2 (**a–c**) Pterygium surgery schematic (**a**) removal of pterygium, (**b**) bare defect, and (**c**) covering of defect with autograft

The Operation

Pterygium surgery involves stripping the pterygium from the cornea and conjunctiva, removing scar tissue from the cornea and the exposed sclera, and finally covering the bare area either with the patient's own conjunctiva harvested from another location or with an amniotic membrane (Fig. 30.2).

Removing the Pterygium

At the start of the surgery, your surgeon may mark the boundary of the pterygium with a gentian violet marker. This serves as a guide during the dissection (Fig. 30.3).

Next, Westcott scissors will be used to make incisions along the border of the pterygium. Your surgeon will then carefully strip the pterygium off the cornea. This

Fig. 30.3 Dissecting
pterygium. (Our
stock image)

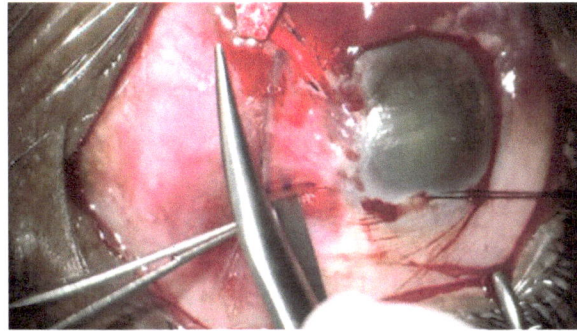

Fig. 30.4 Bare sclera after
dissection. (Our
stock image)

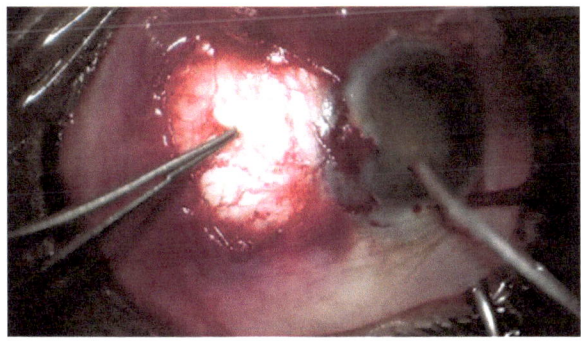

may be done with Westcott scissors, or the pterygium may be avulsed off the cornea surface. To avulse the pterygium head from the cornea, your surgeon will grasp the pterygium neck firmly with 0.12 forceps and forcefully tear off the pterygium head from the cornea using an instrument such as a muscle hook or using the side of any sturdy instrument. If the dissection plane is not perfect when removing the pterygium head or scar tissue has penetrated deeper into the cornea, a 57 blade can be used to create a smoother lamellar dissection. Many surgeons will also use a diamond burr to further polish the cornea surface.

The remaining conjunctival edge of the pterygium will then be dissected off the sclera using Westcott scissors. Many surgeons will dissect all of the Tenon's and scar tissue from the underlying surface of the remaining conjunctival edges. This helps prevent regrowth and provides a better cosmetic appearance once the donor tissue is placed. Typically, a second set of hands either from an assistant or the scrub technician is required. Generally, the assistant elevates the free edges of the conjunctiva with a conjunctival forceps, while the surgeon uses a bond or other fine toothed forceps to dissect the Tenon's tissue off the underside of the free edge of the conjunctiva. The pterygium specimen should be placed in a container with formalin and always sent to pathology. At this point, there will be some amount of bleeding from the remaining scar tissue or the sclera. Your surgeon will use wet field cautery to achieve hemostasis to arrest the bleeding.

Where the pterygium was excised is now a bare area of sclera (Fig. 30.4). If left uncovered, the risk of pterygium recurrence is high; therefore, your surgeon will

Fig. 30.5 Conjunctiva autograft to place over bare sclera. (Our stock image)

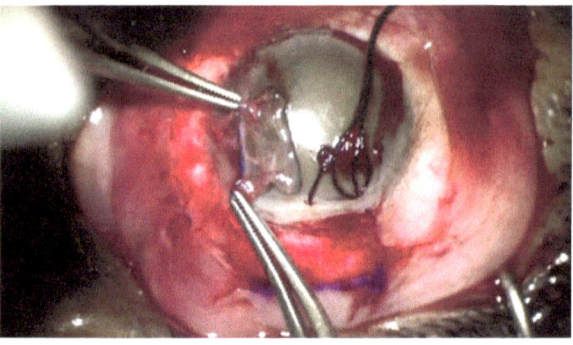

cover the bare area. This may be done using the patient's own conjunctiva harvest from another location in the same eye (termed conjunctival autograft, auto meaning from the patient him/herself) or using a membrane (termed amniotic membrane graft).

Covering the Defect: Using Conjunctival Autograft

A conjunctival autograft is most commonly harvested from the superior (or upper) part of the eye. To expose this part of the eye, often a traction suture consisting of a 4-0 silk or 7-0 Vicryl suture is passed partial thickness through the upper part of the cornea. The ends of the sutures are then pulled down (in the direction toward the patient's feet) and secured to the drape or using a hemostat. This serves to rotate the eye down and expose the upper conjunctiva. Using a gentian violet marker, your surgeon will mark the boundary of the conjunctiva autograft to be harvested. Some surgeon may facilitate the separation of the conjunctiva from the underlying Tenon's fascia by injecting a small amount of epinephrine below the conjunctiva to balloon it.

The dissection begins with Westcott scissors. Your surgeon will then dissect the conjunctiva toward the limbus, leaving the attachment at the limbus last. Finally, the conjunctiva autograft (Fig. 30.5) will be dissected from the limbus.

At this point, your surgeon may remove the traction suture to return the eye to its normal position. The conjunctiva autograft may be secured to the defect left by the pterygium dissection by sutures (typically 10-0 nylon sutures at the limbus and 8-0 Vicryl sutures elsewhere) or more commonly using fibrin-based tissue adhesive such as Tisseel™ fibrin sealant, or a combination of both. Recent literature suggests that pterygium regrowth is much less common when a conjunctival autograft is used than when an amnion membrane is employed.

Fibrin-based tissue adhesives are comprised of two components: human thrombin and a sealer protein solution containing human fibrinogen and aprotinin. When mixed together, the two components combine to mimic the clotting process in human, forming a gel that stop bleeding of wound or allow for adhesion of tissue surface. Tisseel™ fibrin sealant comes in convenient prefilled syringes. Often your surgeon will request the syringes separately, the fibrin containing syringe (thicker) will be given first followed by the sealer protein (thinner) syringe. The mixture quickly coagulates once in contact and allows the graft to be adherent to the defect (Fig. 30.6).

Covering the Defect: Using Amniotic Membrane Graft

In some cases, your surgeon may elect to use an amniotic membrane graft, in lieu of or in adjunct with conjunctival autograft, to cover the defect. An amniotic membrane graft is tissue acquired from the innermost layer of the human placenta and is used to heal damaged mucosal surfaces such as on the eye. It comes in varying sizes and is particularly useful when the defect is large and there is insufficient conjunctival autograft.

Amniotic membrane comes in dual seal pouch. The circulator would open the outer pouch and expos the inner sterile pouch to you. Using sterile non-toothed forceps or your gloved hands, you would grasp the inner pouch that can then be opened over the sterile surgical table (Fig. 30.7). After using scissors to open the pouch, the amniotic membrane graft can be grasped by non-toothed forceps and handed off to the surgeon. Your surgeon will size the amniotic membrane graft to cover the defect and secure it using 8-0 Vicryl sutures or a fibrin-based adhesive such as Tisseel fibrin sealant.

Fig. 30.6 Covering defect with autograft. (Our stock image)

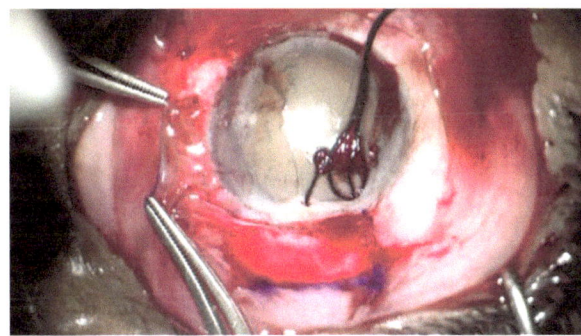

Fig. 30.7 Amniotic membrane graft

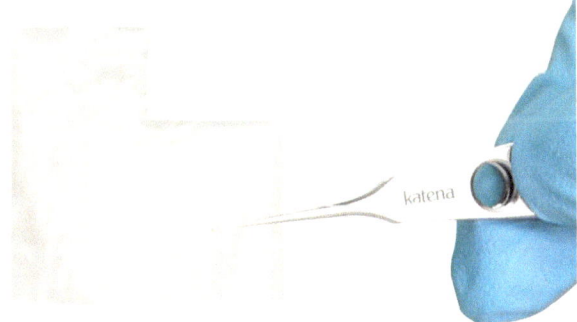

Use of Mitomycin-C

One of the main postoperative events following pterygium surgery is the recurrence of the pterygia. Recurrent pterygia are often more bulky, more vascular, and more difficult to excise than their primary counterparts. They are also associated with a higher rate of recurrence after re-excision. In operating on recurrent pterygium, your surgeon may elect to employ the compound mitomycin-C to reduced recurrence. Mitomycin-C is a natural compound isolated from bacteria. It inhibits DNA synthesis. Mitomycin-C is used in cancer therapy and for the eye, as a topical solution to prevent scar formation. Because it damages DNA, care must be exercised when handling mitomycin-C. All personnel handling the compound must wear protective clothing including gloves, masks, and gown. The sterile surgery clothing is sufficient.

Figure 30.8 shows SuperScrub holding mitomycin.

An OR record should also be kept on the use of mitomycin-C. This includes the strength, the amount of time it was applied to the eye, the lot number from the package, and the number of saturated sponges or Weck-cell sponges placed in and removed from the patient's eye.

If required, mitomycin-C will typically be applied to the defect after the pterygium dissection and before the use of conjunctival autograft or amniotic

Fig. 30.8 Handle mitomycin with care, reminds SuperScrub

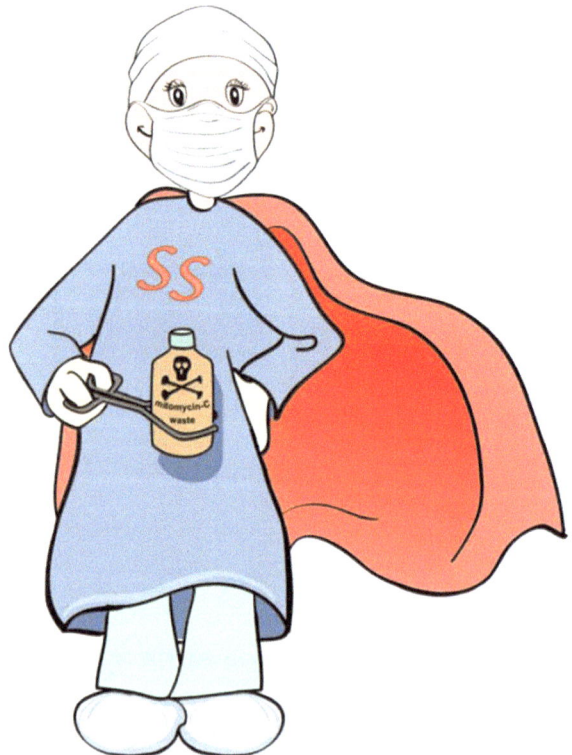

membrane graft. Your surgeon will have decided on the dose of mitomycin-C. Typically, the compound will arrive from your pharmacy in a syringe. Often, to avoid inadvertent application of mitomycin-C to surrounding tissue, your surgeon will ask for Weck-cell sponges dipped in mitomycin-C rather than using the syringe as a dropper. He/she will apply the Weck-cell sponge to the area to be treated. Often only a short duration is required. Your surgeon will indicate to you the duration (typically minutes), and you will inform the surgeon when the time is up. The Weck-cell sponges and the remaining mitomycin-C will then be carefully set aside and discarded following the surgery according to institution guidelines in an appropriate chemotherapy disposal container. If any surgical instrument came in contact with the mitomycin, these too must be set aside and not used on the patient again.

Immediately following the application of the mitomycin-C, your surgeon will copiously irrigate off any residue compound from the eye. The surgical scrub should have several balanced salt solution in 10 cc bottles or a large 30 cc syringe filled with balanced salt solution for this purpose. Use of mitomycin-C has been associated with devastating corneal/scleral melts and infections and therefore should be used judiciously and only for the duration required. The rest of the surgery will proceed with covering of the defect with conjunctival autograft and/or amniotic membrane graft as described above.

Concluding the Case

Pterygium surgery often concludes with application of subconjunctival injection antibiotics and steroid solution. Some surgeons prefer to irrigate the antibiotics onto the ocular surface.

Pterygium Instruments/Supplies

1. Gentian violet marking pen
2. 57 blade
3. Diamond burr
4. 8-0 Vicryl stay suture
5. Westcott scissors
6. Bonn forceps
7. Lid speculum
8. Non-locking needle holder
9. Conjunctival tissue forceps
10. BSS bottles
11. Bipolar cautery

Chapter 31
Band Keratopathy Removal

Band keratopathy is a corneal disease in which calcium deposits on the cornea. It most often occurs in the interpalpebral fissure starting at the nasal and temporal (toward the ear) aspects of the cornea and evolving toward the center, forming a band. Band keratopathy (Fig. 31.1) is often the result of chronic eye inflammation, trauma, or systemic conditions that cause high calcium level such as occurs with kidney failure, certain tumors, and sarcoidosis.

Mild forms of band keratopathy may be observed. Extensive deposits, however, can cause significant irritation or reduced vision if it involves the visual axis. Surgery to remove band keratopathy may be performed in the office at the slit lamp or in the operating room. If performed in the operating room, band keratopathy removal generally requires only MAC sedation and/or topical anesthesia (eye drops).

The Operation

The cornea epithelium needs to be removed to expose the calcium deposits in the deeper Bowman's layer. Your surgeon may request ophthalmic sponges or a blade such as a 57 blade to remove the epithelium. The calcium deposits may be quite recalcitrant to removal; therefore, a solution of 1 M disodium EDTA is often applied after removal of the corneal epithelium. The disodium ethylenediaminetetraacetic acid (EDTA) chelates (binds to) the calcium. The EDTA can be applied directly to the cornea with ophthalmic sponges. Your surgeon will then use a 57 blade to scrape off the calcium. A diamond burr, a round motorized head studded with diamond bits to provide a rough surface, may be used to smooth the surface after the removal of the calcium with the blade. A bandage contact lens, a regular contact lens with no power, will then be placed. The lens will serve to accelerate the healing of the epithelium and eliminate patient discomfort.

© Springer Nature Switzerland AG 2020
R. S. Koplin et al., *The Scrub's Bible*,
https://doi.org/10.1007/978-3-030-44345-0_31

Fig. 31.1 Band
keratopathy. (Our
stock image)

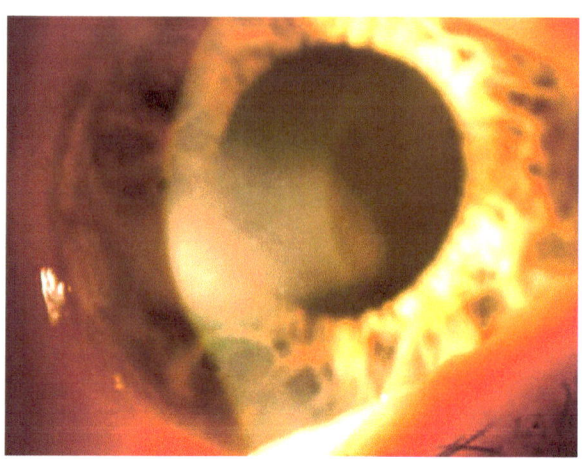

Instruments/supplies

1. 57 blade
2. Wired lid speculum
3. Ophthalmic sponges
4. EDTA (0.5–1.5%) (disodium ethylenediaminetetraacetic acid)
5. Diamond burr
6. Shot glass
7. Bandage contact lens 14-0 mm Plano
8. BSS bottles

Chapter 32
Complications Encountered, Instruments at the Ready: Here Is a List of "What Ifs" and "What to Do's"

During a case of penetrating keratoplasty, your surgeon has removed the patient's cornea button and is about to suture on the donor cornea. The patient coughs and your surgeon notices sudden loss of the red reflex. An expanding dark suprachoroidal mass is noted with expulsion of the intraocular lens.

This is a potentially devastating complication termed an expulsive or suprachoroidal hemorrhage. Risk factors for the occurrence of a suprachoroidal hemorrhage include high intraocular pressure, high blood pressure, old patient age, cardiovascular disease, and sudden decrease of intraocular pressure. For example, when the patient's cornea button is removed, during trephination the eye loses pressure. If the intraocular pressure in the eye was uncontrolled prior to removal of the corneal button, the dramatic decompression can lead to shearing of the choroidal vessels and result in hemorrhage into the suprachoroidal space. The space occupying hemorrhage will lead to progressive increased in pressure and if severe enough can lead to devastating expulsion of intraocular contents, including the lens, vitreous, and even retina, through the open cornea. Sudden increases in eye pressure can also occur with patient movement such as coughing or sneezing or with patient discomfort leading to eye squeezing.

If your surgeon notices an expulsive hemorrhage, he/she will immediately attempt to "close" the eye, that is, suture the donor cornea expeditiously. Your task is to be prepared with sutures and be ready to hand off any required instruments as quickly as possible.

After the donor cornea is secured in place, your surgeon may ask for a #15 blade or an MVR blade (typically used by retinal surgeons to enter the back of the eye) in order to make a stab incision just in front of the retinal insertion at the pars plana (a few millimeters behind the lens and a portion of the anatomy safe to invade). This maneuver by the surgeon is an attempt to divert the increasing choroidal hemorrhage to outside of the eye from behind the choroid, thus diminishing the effect of the blood pushing the choroid and retina out of the eye through the surgical wound(s).

© Springer Nature Switzerland AG 2020
R. S. Koplin et al., *The Scrub's Bible*,
https://doi.org/10.1007/978-3-030-44345-0_32

During a case of endothelial keratoplasty, your surgeon has placed the donor lamella cornea in the patient's anterior chamber. He/she injects air bubble to promote adherence of the donor to the patient's cornea. Suddenly, the anterior chamber becomes flat with iris pushed up against the cornea, the cornea becomes cloudy, and air is noted to be behind the iris.

This is a condition termed pupillary block. Occasionally, during an endothelial keratoplasty procedure, the air migrates behind the iris instead of staying in front. This may occur due to abnormal iris anatomy, excessive air instillation, or without risk factors. The air becomes trapped behind the iris diaphragm, pushing it anteriorly against the cornea. This leads to an increase in intraocular eye, a "hard" eye to palpitation, and patient discomfort.

Your surgeon will immediately release the pupillary block by removing air from behind the iris, typically with a 27 gauge cannula or 30 gauge needle. Following removal of air, the iris will immediately fall back to its normal position and the intraocular pressure normalizes. Surgery can then resume, usually without consequences.

During a case of endothelial keratoplasty, your surgeon has placed the donor lamella cornea in the patient's anterior chamber and is filling the eye with balanced salt solution. Air has not been placed yet. The anterior chamber shallows and the iris is noted to be pushed up against the cornea. The eye feels firm.

Shallowing of the anterior chamber with increase in intraocular pressure can occur due to suprachoroidal hemorrhage or aqueous misdirection. In the first case, a progressive hemorrhage in the suprachoroidal space causes increase in intraocular pressure and pushes intraocular contents forward, causing shallowing of the anterior chamber and elevation in pressure. This is much more common in open globe surgeries like a penetrating keratoplasty and unusual in a small incision surgery like endothelial keratoplasty. In aqueous misdirection, infused saline is "misdirected" behind the lens and trapped in the space between the lens and vitreous (termed anterior hyaloid). This too causes elevation in pressure and shallowing of the anterior chamber. Your surgeon should be able to differentiate between the two causes intraoperatively.

If aqueous misdirection is suspected, as a diagnostic step, your surgeon may perform an iridectomy (an opening in the peripheral iris). If there is any component of pupillary block (where the pupil opening is blocked due to lens or vitreous and preventing the circulation of aqueous fluid), the iridectomy will allow for direct flow of aqueous fluid between the posterior chamber and the anterior chamber, thereby bypassing the pupillary block. To fashion an iridectomy, your surgeon may puncture the peripheral iris by entering through peripheral cornea with a 25 gauge needle, or through a paracentesis, grasp a small tuft of peripheral iris, and create a small opening with Vannas scissors. If pupillary block is the mechanism of shallow anterior chamber, following the iridectomy, aqueous can flow freely and the shallow anterior chamber should resolve. If, however, there continues to be shallow anterior chamber, likely aqueous misdirection is present. If aqueous misdirection is present, your surgeon may request a MVR blade to enter the vitreous via the pars plana to release some vitreous. Drugs such as acetazolamide or mannitol may be administered intravenously to lower the intraocular pressure. If aqueous misdirection is relieved, your surgeon may be able to resume the surgery.

Chapter 33
Surgical Tray: Penetrating Keratoplasty

Corneal Prep Tray: Measures 2 ½ feet by 4 feet – is covered with a sterile plastic backed absorbent sheet.

Prep tray instruments:
1. Moria disposable suction trephine for donor punch
2. Corneal tissue in Krolman viewing chamber
3. 2 × 5 cc syringe (one for suction trephination and one for Optisol-GS solution)
4. Toothed tissue forceps to grasp donor tissue

Surgical tray instruments:
1. Flieringa rings set
2. Closed loop wire lid speculum
3. RK marker (12 and 16)
4. Gentian violet marking pen
5. 1 diamond paracentesis blade or 15 degree metal blade
6. 1 Westcott scissors
7. 1 Vannas scissors
8. Corneal scissors (left and right)
9. 1 0.12 toothed forceps
10. 1 0.3 toothed forceps
11. 1 Girard forceps or 1 Colibri forceps
12. Tennant tying forceps: straight and curved
13. 1 Kelman style forceps – toothed
14. 1 Kelman style forceps – non-toothed
15. Two needle holders: locking and non-locking
16. 1 cyclodialysis spatula
17. 1 Paton tissue spatula
18. Package of ophthalmic sponges (10)
19. 1 3 cc syringe + blunt 27 gauge cannula filled with BSS
20. 1 vial of viscoelastic

© Springer Nature Switzerland AG 2020
R. S. Koplin et al., *The Scrub's Bible*,
https://doi.org/10.1007/978-3-030-44345-0_33

21. 10 cc BSS bottles to moisten cornea
22. 1 empty 3 cc syringe (swing)
23. Surgeon's and assistant's sterile gloves
24. Surgeon's gown
25. Disposable identification stickers to be applied to various injectables
26. Needles – 10-0 Nylon on Alcon CU-5 needle or Ethicon C-160 needle

Standby items:
1. 10-0 Prolene on C160-6 for pupilloplasty
2. Anterior vitrectomy setup if vitreous in anterior chamber
3. Kuglen and Sinisky hooks if IOL manipulation

Chapter 34
Surgical Tray: Keratoprosthesis

Corneal Prep Tray: Measures 2 ½ feet by 4 feet – is covered with a sterile plastic backed absorbent sheet.

Prep Tray Instruments:
1. Moria disposable suction trephine for donor punch
2. Corneal tissue in Krolman viewing chamber
3. 2 × 5 cc syringe (one for suction trephination and one for Optisol-GS solution)
4. Toothed tissue forceps to grasp donor tissue

Surgical Tray Instruments:
1. Flieringa rings set
2. Fixation ring
3. Closed loop wire lid speculum
4. RK marker (12 and 16)
5. Gentian violet marking pen
6. 1 Diamond paracentesis blade or 15 degree blade
7. 1 Westcott scissors
8. 1 Vannas scissors
9. Corneal scissors (left and right)
10. 1 0.12 forceps
11. 1 0.3 forceps
12. 1 Colibri forceps or 1 Girard forceps
13. Tennant tying forceps: straight and curved
14. 1 Kelman style forceps – toothed
15. 1 Kelman style forceps – non-toothed
16. Two needle holders: locking and non-locking
17. 1 cyclodialysis spatula
18. 1 tissue spatula
19. Package of ophthalmic sponges (10) (Weck-cells)
20. 1 3 cc syringe + blunt 27 gauge cannula filled with BSS

© Springer Nature Switzerland AG 2020
R. S. Koplin et al., *The Scrub's Bible*,
https://doi.org/10.1007/978-3-030-44345-0_34

21. 1 vial of viscoelastic
22. 1 empty 3 cc syringe (swing)
23. Surgeon's and assistant's sterile gloves
24. Surgeon's gown
25. Disposable identification stickers to be applied to various injectables
26. Needles – 10-0 Nylon on Alcon CU-5 needle or Ethicon C-160 needle

Standby Items:
1. 10-0 prolene on C160-6 for pupilloplasty
2. Anterior vitrectomy setup if vitreous in anterior chamber
3. Kuglen and Sinisky hooks if IOL manipulation

1. 1 0.3 forceps
2. Additional Colibri forceps or 1 Girard forceps
3. Tennant tying forceps: straight and curved
4. 1 Kelman style forceps – toothed
5. 1 Kelman style forceps – non-toothed
6. Two needle holders: locking and non -locking
7. 1 cyclodialysis spatula
8. 1 Paton tissue spatula
9. Package of mini-cellulose sponges (10) (Weck-cells)
10. 1 3 cc syringe + blunt 27 gauge cannula filled with BSS
11. 1 vial of viscoelastic
12. 10 cc BSS bottles to moisten cornea
13. 1 empty 3 cc syringe (swing)
14. Surgeon's and assistant's sterile gloves
15. Surgeon's gowns
16. Disposable identification stickers to be applied to various injectables

Sutures
1. Needles – 10-0 Nylon on Alcon CU-5 needle or Ethicon C-160 needle

Standby Items:
1. 10-0 Prolene on C160-6 for pupilloplasty
2. Anterior vitrectomy setup if vitreous in anterior chamber
3. Kuglen and Sinisky hooks if IOL manipulation

Chapter 35
Surgical Tray: DSAEK

Corneal Prep Tray: Measures 2 ½ feet by 4 feet – is covered with a sterile plastic backed absorbent sheet.

Prep Tray Instruments:
1. Moria disposable suction trephine for donor punch
2. Corneal tissue in Krolman viewing chamber
3. 2 × 5 cc syringe (one for suction trephination and one for Optisol-GS solution)
4. Toothed tissue forceps to grasp donor tissue

Surgical Tray Instruments:
1. Anterior chamber maintainer connected to IV pole
2. Closed loop wire lid speculum
3. 8 or 9 mm optic zone marker
4. Gentian violet marking pen
5. 1 diamond paracentesis blade or 15 degree blade
6. 1 diamond keratome or metal keratome blade (2.75–3.0 mm)
7. 1 0.12 forceps
8. 1 0.3 forceps
9. 1 Colibri forceps or 1 Girard forceps
10. Tennant tying forceps: straight and curved
11. 1 Kelman style forceps: toothed
12. 1 Kelman style forceps – non-toothed
13. Two needle holders: locking and non-locking
14. 1 Reverse Sinskey hook (Endoscorer)
15. 1 Endothelial stripper
16. 1 Metal keratome (2.75–3.0 mm)
17. 1 Westcott scissors
18. 1 Vannas scissors
19. 1 Endothelial inserter (mini-Busin glide or Coronet EndoGlide)
20. Package of mini-cellulose sponges (10) (Weck-cells)

© Springer Nature Switzerland AG 2020
R. S. Koplin et al., *The Scrub's Bible*,
https://doi.org/10.1007/978-3-030-44345-0_35

21. 1 1 cc syringe + 27 gauge blunt cannula containing 1% lidocaine injectable
22. 1 3 cc syringe + blunt 27 gauge cannula filled with BSS
23. 1 empty 3 cc syringe (for air)
24. 10 cc BSS bottles to moisten cornea
25. 1 50 cc bottle of sterile balanced salt solution (BSS). (This can be supplied as a factory prepared bottle or as sterile squeeze bottle that can be filled multiple times from protected, capped, bottles of IV saline.)
26. Surgeon's and assistant's sterile gloves
27. Surgeon's gowns

Sutures:
1. 10-0 Nylon on Alcon CU-5 or Ethicon 160-0 Needle

Optional Supplies:
1. Miochol™ or Miostat™ for papillary miosis
2. SF_6 Gas Canister with 10 cc syringe and filter

Chapter 36
Surgical Tray: DMEK

Corneal Prep Tray It measures 2½ feet by 4 feet and is covered with a sterile plastic backed absorbent sheet.

Prep Tray Instruments
1. Prestained, premarked corneal tissue scrolled in modified Jones Straiko tube inside a Krolman viewing chamber
2. Hemostat to grasp modified Jones Straiko Glass Tube
3. Petri dish filled with BSS solution
4. 14 French precut catheter tubing attached to a 5 cc syringe

Surgical Tray Instruments
1. Sinskey hook (Katena Instruments)
2. Kuglen Hook
3. Gentian violet marking pen
4. Straiko Modified Glass Jones tube (Gunther Weiss Scientific Glassblowing Co., Portland, Oregon)
5. 14 French tubing with male and female adaptors
6. 5 cc syringe filled with BSS
7. 10 cc BSS bottles to moisten the cornea
8. Diamond or metal keratome (2.4–2.8 mm)
9. Reverse Sinskey hook (Moria)
10. Descemet stripper (Moria)
11. 8 or 9 mm optical zone marker (Moria)
12. Anterior chamber maintainer connected to IV pole
13. Closed-loop wire lid speculum
14. 1 diamond paracentesis blade or 15 degree blade
15. 1 diamond keratome or metal keratome blade (2.75–3.0 mm)
16. 1 0.12 forceps
17. 1 Colibri forceps or 1 Girard forceps
18. Tennant tying forceps: straight and curved

© Springer Nature Switzerland AG 2020
R. S. Koplin et al., *The Scrub's Bible*,
https://doi.org/10.1007/978-3-030-44345-0_36

19. Fine needle holders: non-locking
20. Package of mini-cellulose ophthalmic sponges (10)
21. 1 1 cc syringe + 27 gauge blunt cannula containing 1% lidocaine injectable
22. 1 3 cc syringe + blunt 27 gauge cannula filled with BSS
23. 1 empty 3 cc syringe (for air)
24. Surgeon's and assistant sterile gloves
25. Surgeon's gowns

Sutures
1. 10-0 nylon on Alcon CU-5 or Ethicon 160-0 needle

Optional Supplies
1. Miochol®-E (acetylcholine) or Miostat® (carbachol 0.01%) for papillary miosis
2. SF_6 gas canister with 10 cc syringe and filter

Chapter 37
Surgical Tray Pterygium

1. Gentian violet marking pen
2. 57 blade
3. Westcott scissors (sharp/blunt)
4. Iris Wills conjunctival tissue forceps
5. Bonn forceps
6. Lid speculum
7. Heavy locking needle holder
8. Diamond burr

Additional Supplies
1. 7-0 silk (stay suture to rotate eye)
2. Non-locking needle holder
3. Bipolar cautery with eraser tip
4. Tisseel™ fibrin adhesive
5. Amniotic membrane graft (AmnioGraft™ Biotissue, Miami, Florida)
6. 8-0 Vicryl suture (prn for additional fixation)
7. 1% lidocaine with epinephrine on 5 cc syringe (prn extra anesthesia)

© Springer Nature Switzerland AG 2020   199
R. S. Koplin et al., *The Scrub's Bible*,
https://doi.org/10.1007/978-3-030-44345-0_37

Chapter 38
Self-Assessment Test for Corneal Surgery

1. True or False: The cornea consists of three layers: the outer epithelium which provides protection against infection, injury, and desiccation; the central stroma which consists of fibers that provide strength; and the inner endothelium which contains cells that pump fluid out of the cornea to maintain transparency.

   Answer: True.

2. True or False: Damage to the corneal layers from causes such as infection, inflammation, and trauma can lead to loss of corneal clarity and always require surgery to restore vision.

   Answer: False. While damage to the corneal layers can lead to loss of clarity, surgery is only considered when the damage causes irreversible loss of vision. In some cases, the damage is peripheral and does not interfere with vision. In some, medical therapy may be used to reverse the damage.

3. True or False: Retrobulbar anesthesia requires a short (5/8 inch) needle.

   Answer: False. Retrobulbar anesthesia is delivered deep into the space behind the eye and therefore requires a longer (1.5 inch) needle.

4. True or False: Penetrating keratoplasty is surgery that involves replacement of selective layers of the cornea, while endothelial keratoplasty involves replacement of the entire thickness of the cornea.

   Answer: False. As its name implies, *penetrating* keratoplasty penetrates and hence involves the entire thickness of the cornea. *Endothelial* keratoplasty involves replacement of only the endothelium and the deep stromal layers.

5. True or False: In penetrating keratoplasty, the patient's cornea is removed free hand by the surgeon so that any shape can be fashioned.

   Answer: False. A circular trephine (a metal tubular device with sharp blade at one end) is used in corneal transplant surgery. This allows for precise circular shape and size to be fashioned. Similarly, the donor cornea is cut using a trephine to match the patient's trephination. As scrub technician, you may be required to obtain these trephines for your surgeons.

© Springer Nature Switzerland AG 2020
R. S. Koplin et al., *The Scrub's Bible*,
https://doi.org/10.1007/978-3-030-44345-0_38

6. True or False: During keratoplasty surgery, confirm the type and size of trephines verbally prior to opening them.
   Answer: True. Using a trephine of the wrong size can lead to inaccurate siz-
ing of the transplant which in turn can lead to difficulty in closing the surgical wound.

7. Order the following steps in penetrating keratoplasty surgery:

   (a) Trephination of donor cornea
   (b) Placing marks for suture placement (optional)
   (c) Securing a Flieringa ring to the episclera (optional)
   (d) Trephination of patient cornea
   (e) Securing donor cornea to patient's eye with sutures

   Answer: c, b, a, d, e.

8. True or False: In keratoplasty surgery, the donor cornea is handled in a sterile
fashion. The circulator opens the container over a sterile side table and the surgeon then grasps the cornea with sterile instruments.
   Answer: True.

9. Which of the following instrument is used to bury sutures:

   (a) 0.12 forceps
   (b) Colibri forceps
   (c) 0.3 forceps
   (d) Tying forceps

   Answer: d. A non-toothed forceps, in particular the tying forceps, is used to
bury knots. Toothed forceps such as 0.12 and 0.3 forceps (the larger the number
the coarser the tip) are used to grasp tissue; their sharp teeth will tear sutures
and therefore are not used in burying sutures. Colibri forceps are also toothed
forceps.

10. Which of the following is true regarding "open sky" (when the patient's cornea
has been removed during keratoplasty and the eye is "open")?

   (a) This exposes the patient to the risk of expulsive hemorrhage.
   (b) Any patient movement is discouraged until the donor cornea is secured
       in placed.
   (c) Your surgeon will work expeditiously to secure the donor cornea in place.

   Answer: All of the above.

11. True or False: In keratoprosthesis surgery, a donor cornea is not required.
   Answer: False. Although the keratoprosthesis is an artificial cornea made of
plastic material, the cornea from a deceased donor tissue is still required. This
donor cornea will be sandwiched between the front plate and back plate of the
keratoprosthesis assembly.

12. True or False: The surgical steps of keratoprosthesis surgery are similar to the
steps of penetrating keratoplasty, aside from the preparation of the donor cornea (in keratoprosthesis surgery, a central 3 mm hole is fashioned) and assembly of keratoprosthesis.
   Answer: True.

13. True or False: In Descemet stripping automated endothelial keratoplasty (DSAEK), the eye bank will fashion the donor lenticule with a microkeratome to create the posterior lamella (layer of cornea consisting of Descemet's membrane and posterior stroma) and then replace the anterior lenticule so that the tissue arrives precut to the operating room.

    Answer: True.

14. True or False: In DSEK and DMEK, the entire thickness of the patient's cornea is removed.

    Answer: False. In DSAEK and DMEK, only the Descemet's membrane of the patient's cornea is removed. The surgeon typically removed the membrane using a reverse Sinskey hook and an endothelial stripper.

15. True or False: In DMEK, the donor cornea comes prestained and prefolded into a modified Jones Straiko glass tube, ready for insertion without surgeon manipulation of the tissue.

    Answer: True.

16. True or False: At the conclusion of DMEK or DSAEK, the patient is free to sit up and resume normal activities.

    Answer: False: Following DMEK or DSAEK, the patient is instructed to remain flat (except for necessary short breaks) usually until the next day so that the air bubble can tamponade the donor cornea against the patient's cornea, promoting adherence.

17. True or False: In pterygium surgery, the defect following removal of the pterygium can be left bare exposing the sclera.

    Answer: False. Leaving the area of pterygium excision bare greatly increases the risk of recurrence of the pterygium. Therefore, the defect is either covered with conjunctival autograft or amniotic membrane graft.

18. True or False: The excised pterygium can be discarded at the end of surgery.

    Answer: False. Any specimen from the patient, be it pterygium or cornea button, must be placed in a container (usually with formalin) to send to pathology department for analysis.

19. True or False: Amniotic membrane graft is tissue acquired from the innermost layer of the human placenta and is used to heal damaged mucosal surfaces such as on the eye.

    Answer: True.

20. True or False: Tisseel™ glue is made up of the same material contained in Krazy Glue™ (cyanoacrylate).

    Answer: False. Tisseel glue is comprised of two components: human thrombin and a sealer protein consisting of human fibrinogen and aprotonin. These are involved in the human clotting process. Tisseel glue is used in eye surgery to achieve hemostasis and for tissue adherence.

21. Proper ways to handle mitomycin-C includes all of the following except:

    (a) Discarding mitomycin-C soaked sponges and Weck-cells in chemical disposal container.

    (b) Wearing protective clothing such as surgical gown, masks, and gloves.

(c) Instruments that came in contact with the mitomycin-C can be reused at a later step during the same surgery.

(d) Irrigating the eye copiously following use of mitomycin-C.

Answer: c. Instruments that can in contact with mitomycin-C should be set aside, not to be reused in the same surgery, to be cleaned and sterilized.

22. True or False: Mitomycin-C is genotoxic (damages DNA) and must be handled with care.

Answer: True.

23. Documentation for mitomycin-C use includes:

(a) Strength (i.e., concentration)

(b) Amount of time it was applied to the eye

(c) Lot number from the package

(d) Number of saturated sponges or ophthalmic sponges placed in and removed from the patient's eye

Answer: All of the above.

24. You noticed that a ophthalmic sponge soaked with mitomycin-C is unaccounted for. You should:

(a) Assume the ophthalmic sponge has mostly likely fallen into the side drape and is unlikely to remain tucked around the patient's eye.

(b) If still on the eye, assume the ophthalmic sponge will likely fall out on its own following the surgery.

(c) Notify your surgeon so that the ophthalmic sponge can be found and is accounted for.

Answer: c. Nothing that comes into contact with mitomycin-C should remain in the patient's eye. Exposure to mitomycin-C can be associated with scleral and corneal melt.

25. True or False: A solution of calcium EDTA may be used to remove band keratopathy.

Answer: False. Band keratopathy is calcium deposits in the cornea. Removal requires use of disodium (not calcium) EDTA.

26. True or False: At the conclusion of any surgery, ensure that all needles used are accounted for.

Answer: True.

27. All of the following are effective measures to prevent needle stick injuries in ophthalmology except:

(a) Neutral zone (hands free technique) needle passage

(b) Operating room education and inservices

(c) Blunt tip suture needles

(d) Following standard procedures, infection prevention and general hygiene practices

Answer: c. Although blunt tip sutures needles have drastically reduced needle sticks in many surgical specialties, they do not work well with ocular tissue.

Chapter 39
Resource Materials

The following offer information relevant to the needs of Scrub Technologists and Scrub Nurses:

Web Portals

American Society of Ophthalmic Registered Nurses (ASORN)
https://asorn.org/ Fosters excellence in ophthalmic patient care while supporting both ophthalmic registered nurse and technicians through evidence based practice.

Association of periOperative Registered Nurses (AORN)
https://www.aorn.org/ Excellent site for general perioperative practice information.
  Utilizes evidence-based data providing the reader through Perioperative Standards and Recommended Practices for the RN and Scrub Technician.

Association of Surgical Technologists (AST)
https://www.ast.org/ Association and Certification standards are determined state to state to ensure that surgical technologists have the knowledge and skill to administer patient care of the highest quality. Information on more than 40 state organizations of continuing education for surgical technologists.

EyeWiki
https://eyewiki.aao.org/Main_Page Free online ophthalmic encyclopedia that covers the vast spectrum of eye disease, diagnosis, and treatment. Includes hundreds of articles written by ophthalmologists.

© Springer Nature Switzerland AG 2020
R. S. Koplin et al., *The Scrub's Bible*,
https://doi.org/10.1007/978-3-030-44345-0_39

Additional Clinical Education Resources

Books

Ophthalmic Procedures in the Operating Room and Ambulatory Surgery Center, 4th Edition Print book for all operating room staff includes objectives, step-by-step instructions, and a list of equipment and instruments required for a variety of surgical procedures. Published by ASORN. Available at https://store.aao. org/ophthalmic-procedures-in-the-operating-room-and-ambulatory-surgery-center-fourth-edition.html

Care and Handling of Ophthalmic Microsurgical Instruments, 4th Edition Print book that outlines in detail the correct methods for sterilizing, storing, and maintaining instruments used in an ophthalmic practice. Published by ASORN. Available at https://store.aao.org/care-and handling-of-ophthalmic-microsurgical-instruments-fourth-edition.html

Chapter 40
Glossary of Terms

Anterior chamber (AC) space behind cornea and in front of iris, filled with aqueous humor.

Anterior chamber intraocular lens (ACIOL) synthetic lens placed in the anterior chamber during cataract surgery to replace the crystalline lens.

Aqueous humor fluid occupying the anterior chamber; maintains intraocular eye pressure and provides eye tissues with nutrients.

Biometry the process of measuring the power of the cornea (keratometry) and the length of the eye, and using the data to determine the ideal intraocular lens power.

Band keratopathy a corneal condition where calcium deposits in the Bowman's layer causing irritation or reduced vision.

Capsule thin glassine-like lining surrounding the nucleus and cortex of the crystalline lens.

Cataract clouded crystalline lens due to age and medical conditions such as diabetes, trauma, and steroid use; causes reduced vision.

Choroid vascular tissue between the retina and the sclera which supplies nutrients to the retina.

Ciliary body muscle/vascular structure within the eye and sits at approximately the level of the lens. It connects the choroid (in the back of the eye) to the iris (in front of the eye); it produces aqueous humor (the fluid that fills the front of the eye).

Ciliary sulcus valley between the iris and ciliary body and circling the eye; a handy anatomical spot, to place an intraocular lens implant when it cannot be placed safely in the capsular bag.

Conjunctiva lubricating mucous membrane lining most of the front of the eye (sclera) and the under surface of eyelids.

Continuous curvilinear capsulorrhexis (CCC, rhexis) the making of a continuous circular tear in the anterior capsule during cataract surgery in order to allow access to the nucleus and cortex.

Cornea transparent dome-shaped tissue vaulting the very front of the eye; allows for transmission of light; provides most of the focusing power of the eye.

© Springer Nature Switzerland AG 2020
R. S. Koplin et al., *The Scrub's Bible*,
https://doi.org/10.1007/978-3-030-44345-0_40

Crystalline lens biconvex transparent lens structure behind the iris and in front of the vitreous; together with the cornea, contributes to focusing power of the eye.

Descemet stripping automated endothelial keratoplasty (DSAEK) a partial thickness corneal transplant surgery in which descemets membrane and the diseased endothelium of the cornea are replaced with a healthy donor cornea lenticule (consisting of endothelium and between 80 and 120 microns of posterior stroma.

Descemet membrane endothelial keratoplasty (DMEK) a partial thickness corneal transplant surgery in which the diseased descemet membrane and endothelium of the cornea is removed and replaced with healthy donor cornea endothelium and descemet membrane without additional stromal tissue from the donor.

Endothelium (Endo) innermost layer of the cornea facing the anterior chamber; comprises of cells that continuously pump fluid out of the cornea to keep it transparent.

Epithelium (Epi) outermost layer of the cornea; provides protection against injury, infection, and desiccation.

Extended depth of focus IOLs (EDF or EDOF) a new type of multifocal intraocular lens (IOL) technology designed to allow for an extended range of sharp vison and a lower incidence of halos and glare than seen in many other multifocal IOLs.

Extracapsular cataract extraction (ECCE) cataract surgery in which the cataractous lens is removed in one piece; requires large incision and sutures.

Extraocular muscle muscles that control eye movement.

Femtosecond laser-assisted cataract surgery (FLACS) an advanced type of cataract surgery that uses femtosecond laser technology to provide a high level of precision to specific steps in the surgery that traditionally have been performed with handheld surgical tools. These steps include the corneal incision, the anterior capsulotomy, and lens fragmentation.

Fovea a small depression in the center of the macula where the visual acuity is the highest. The center of the field of vision is focused in this region.

Haptic an arm of the lens implant that extends from the lens itself at either end and shaped like an "elbow" of sorts. Haptics are lens stabilizers, and it is important that they are not damaged in handling.

Hydrodissection a step in cataract surgery in which the lens capsule is separated from the lens cortex with the use of balanced salt solution (BSS) on a syringe to free any adhesions between the capsule and the cortex.

Intraocular floppy iris syndrome (IFIS) a complication that may occur during cataract surgery. It is characterized by a flaccid or floppy iris which billows in response to normal intraocular currents causing the iris to prolapse into the cataract wound and the pupil to constrict during surgery.

Intracapsular cataract extraction (ICCE) cataract surgery in which the cataractous lens is removed in its entirety including the lens capsule.

Intraocular lens (IOL) synthetic lens inserted during cataract surgery to replace the crystalline lens; can be placed in the capsular bag, ciliary sulcus, or anterior chamber or sewn onto the iris or sclera.

Intraocular pressure (IOP) pressure exerted by fluid within the eye. When inordinately high can cause glaucoma and damage to the optic nerve of the eye. This can lead to blindness.

Iris pigmented muscular tissue between the cornea and the crystalline lens that regulates the amount of light entering the eye by affecting the size of the pupil. If you are familiar with old-fashioned cameras, consider that the pupil acts as a diaphragm to regulate the amount of light entering the eye.

Irrigation and aspiration (IA or I&A) refers to the dual function of infusing fluid into the eye (irrigation) and removing fluid along with any lens or cortical material from the eye (aspiration); a vital process during cataract surgery.

Keratoprosthesis (KPro) an artificial cornea made of plastic material, utilized in corneal transplant surgery when donor cornea is thought to carry high risk of subsequent transplant failure.

Lacrimal gland gland located in the upper outer portion of the orbit that produces tears.

Lens implant a plastic or silicone lens usually smaller than the head of a small thumb-tack; often soft and flexible and fabricated from a single piece of plastic; occasionally three pieces: one lens and two haptics.

Limbus boundary between cornea and sclera, a surgical landmark.

Macula pigmented yellow area near the center of the retina; contains structures for fine vision perception.

Microinvasive glaucoma surgery (MIGS) a class of microsurgical techniques occasionally used in conjunction with cataract surgery to lower intraocular pressure, which have less risk, with fewer complications, than other more invasive glaucoma surgery techniques.

MiLoop is a lens fragmentation device which uses micro-thin, super-elastic, self-expanding nitinol filament technology to fragment cataractous lenses especially in very dense cataracts.

Multifocal IOLs (MFIOLs) a type of intraocular lens (IOL) designed to provide focus of both distance and near objects.

Optic nerve bundle of nerve fibers that transmits electrical signal from the eye to the brain.

Optiwave refractive analysis (ORA) a technology which uses wavefront analysis of the eye to improve accuracy and provide better outcomes in cataract surgery. The device attaches to the operating room microscope and provides intraoperative biometry measurements to help calculate intraocular lens power.

Orbit boney socket containing the eyeball, optic nerve, extraocular muscles, fat, blood vessels, and nerves.

Pars plana area of inner eye approximately behind iris and retina which is free of important structures and considered an ideal place to enter the eye for surgery of the vitreous or retina.

Pars plana lensectomy (PPL) a surgical technique wherein the entire lens (anterior capsule, cortex, nucleus, and posterior capsule) is removed using pars plana sclerotomy ports.

Penetrating keratoplasty corneal surgery in which full thickness of patient's diseased cornea is replaced with healthy donor cornea.

Peribulbar anesthetic injection anesthetic injection given around the orbit using a short needle; this avoids the deeper structures in the orbit.

Phacoemulsification process in which the crystalline lens is broken into small pieces by ultrasound to facilitate removal of the lens through a small incision.

Posterior chamber (PC) space behind iris and in front of the crystalline lens, filled with aqueous humor.

Posterior chamber intraocular lens (PCIOL) synthetic lens inserted in the posterior chamber (in capsular bag, ciliary sulcus, or sewn or glued into the iris or sclera) during cataract surgery to replace the crystalline lens.

Pterygium wing-shaped benign growth from the conjunctiva onto the cornea; can cause irritation or reduced vision.

Pupil circular opening in the center of the iris that allows light to enter the eye; movement of the iris changes the size of the pupil.

Retina multilayered sensory tissue that lines the inside wall of the eye; contains light-sensing cells that convert light into electrical signals which travel to the brain via the optic nerve.

Retrobulbar anesthetic injection anesthetic injection given deep into the orbit below the eyeball (globe) using a long needle; allows for long-duration anesthesia and causes akinesia (lack of eye movement) in addition to anesthesia.

Sclera white fibrous protective outer covering of the eye.

Stroma middle thickest layer of the cornea comprised of collagen fibers.

Trephine surgical instrument with a circular blade used to cut cornea during corneal transplant surgery.

Trifocal IOLs a type of multifocal IOL used to focus images clearly onto the retina at both near, intermediate, and distance and thus reduce the need for glasses after cataract surgery.

Vitreous transparent jelly-like substance between the crystalline lens and the retina.

Zonule fibrous strands that extend from the ciliary body to the crystalline lens suspending it.

Chapter 41
Medications List

Here you will find a list of the medications commonly used in cataract and corneal surgeries.

Acetazolamide (Diamox)—used to lower intraocular pressure by reducing production of aqueous humor.

Atropine—long-acting mydriatic (dilates the pupil) and cycloplegic (paralyzes the ciliary muscle of the eye, resulting in loss of accommodation which is the process whereby the natural lens of the eye change shape to allow for focusing at different distances); in corneal surgery, it may be used at the conclusion of Descemet stripping endothelial keratoplasty to prevent pupillary block.

Cyclopentolate (Cyclogyl)—a mydriatic and cycloplegic; in corneal surgery, it may be used at the conclusion of Descemet stripping endothelial keratoplasty to prevent pupillary block or used to dilate the pupil to examine children.

Epinephrine—a hormone and neurotransmitter that acts on nearly all body tissues; some of its functions include vasoconstriction (constrict blood vessels), muscle contraction, acceleration of heart, and respiratory rate. As a medication for the eye, it is used in conjunction with local anesthetic such as bupivacaine to increase its duration of action and to reduce bleeding. It is also used as a preservative-free formulation injected into the anterior chamber during cataract surgery to dilate the pupil and prevent floppy iris.

Fentanyl—a narcotic analgesia (medication that blocks pain); used intravenously in conjunction with propofol or midazolam for induction of anesthesia.

Homatropine—an intermediate-acting mydriatic and cycloplegic; in corneal surgery, it may be used at the conclusion of Descemet stripping endothelial keratoplasty to prevent pupillary block.

Hyaluronidase—an enzyme that catalyzes the breakdown of extracellular matrix protein; used in conjunction with peribulbar or retrobulbar anesthetic injection to increase its tissue permeability by breaking down proteins in the extracellular (outside of cell) part of eye tissue.

© Springer Nature Switzerland AG 2020
R. S. Koplin et al., *The Scrub's Bible*,
https://doi.org/10.1007/978-3-030-44345-0_41

Lidocaine—fast-acting anesthetic; used as a preservative-free solution to be injected into anterior chamber during surgery or used as a gel on the surface of the eye.

Marcaine—combination of bupivacaine (long-acting anesthetic) and epinephrine. Bupivacaine is given as peribulbar or retrobulbar injection where longer duration of anesthesia is desired, as in corneal surgery. Epinephrine constricts blood vessels, reducing bleeding associated with the injection, and reduces absorption of the bupivacaine, increasing its duration of action.

Mannitol—a diuretic used to dehydrate the vitreous and thereby reduces intraocular pressure.

Midazolam (Versed)—short-acting drug that has sedative, anxiolytic (relieves anxiety), muscle relaxant, and amnestic (causes patient to not recall the procedure) properties; given intravenously to induce anesthesia.

Miochol (Acetylcholine)—acetylcholine neurotransmitter that acts on the nervous system in the body; used as an injection into the anterior chamber during eye surgery to achieve rapid constriction of the pupil.

Mitomycin-C—compound isolated from bacteria that inhibits DNA synthesis; used on the eye to prevent scar formation.

Phenylephrine (Neosynephrine)—a mydriatic used to dilate the pupil for eye examination or surgery.

Povidine iodine—broad spectrum antiseptic used for prevention of infections; used to prep the patient's eye and face for surgery.

Proparacaine (Alcaine)—short-acting anesthetic used as an eye drop for eye examination or surgery.

Propofol—a short-acting hypnotic agent, given intravenously to induce and maintain anesthesia.

Tetracaine—a short-acting anesthetic used as an eye drop for eye examination or surgery.

Tropicamide—a mydriatic and cycloplegic; used to dilate the pupil and relax accommodation for eye examination or surgery.

Appendix A:
Surgeon Instrument Preferences
Note Cataract Surgery

Dr. X
Kuglen hook
30° phaco tip
IA with soft sleeve
Lidocaine 1% non-preserved
Nagahara chopper
Diamond blade

© Springer Nature Switzerland AG 2020
R. S. Koplin et al., *The Scrub's Bible*,
https://doi.org/10.1007/978-3-030-44345-0

Appendix B:
Patient Identification Wall Note

January 12, 2013
Patient: John Malloy
Date of Birth: 3/22/33
Surgeon: Dr. Y
Right Eye Cataract with Implant

© Springer Nature Switzerland AG 2020
R. S. Koplin et al., *The Scrub's Bible*,
https://doi.org/10.1007/978-3-030-44345-0

Index

© Springer Nature Switzerland AG 2020
R. S. Koplin et al., *The Scrub's Bible*,
https://doi.org/10.1007/978-3-030-44345-0